# Prostate Cancer

*BST*

# Prostate Cancer

EDITED BY

Nadine Jelsing

⩞

*Foreword by*

Jon M. Huntsman Sr.

# Portraits of Empowerment

CONTRIBUTORS

Paul Georgeades

Aarol (Bud) Irish

John Plosnich

Charlie Russ

Virgil Simons

Peter Stults

Manuel Vazquez

Bob White

Derek Workman

Don Zank

Westview Press
A Member of the Perseus Books Group

Copyright © 1999 by Westview Press, A Member of the Perseus Books Group

Published in 1999 in the United States of America by Westview Press, 5500 Central Avenue, Boulder, Colorado 80301-2877, and in the United Kingdom by Westview Press, 12 Hid's Copse Road, Cumnor Hill, Oxford OX2 9JJ


Library of Congress Cataloging-in-Publication Data
Prostate cancer : portraits of empowerment /
   edited by Nadine Jelsing; with a foreword by Jon M. Huntsman Sr.;
contributors Paul Georgeades ... [et al.].
      p.   cm.
   Includes bibliographical references.
   ISBN 0-8133-6657-7
   1. Prostate—Cancer—Popular works.   I. Jelsing, Nadine.
II. Georgeades, Paul.
RC280.P7P7597   1999
616.99'463—dc21                                                        98-45154
                                                                            CIP


The paper used in this publication meets the requirements of the American National Standard for Permanence of Paper for Printed Library Materials Z39.48-1984.

10   9   8   7   6   5   4   3   2   1

*To all the men and their families who are battling
prostate cancer now and to all those who
will face that battle in the future*

# Contents

*Foreword*, Jon M. Huntsman Sr.                                     ix
*Preface*                                                           xiii
*Acknowledgments*                                                   xvi
*About the Contributors*                                            xvii

1   Diagnosis: A Change in Priorities                               1

2   Decisions: The Learning Curve                                   25

3   Your Health Care Team: A Proactive Approach                     63

4   Treatments: Action and Recovery                                 79

5   Living with Prostate Cancer                                     107

6   Sex, Love, and Intimacy                                         143

7   A Woman's Point of View: The Wives' Stories                     161

8   Money Talk: Insurance and Finances                              173

9   Recurrence: Strategies for Survival                             189

10  Advocacy and Education: Toward a Cure                           217

11  Hindsight and Future Visions: Philosophies Revisited            239

*Epilogue*                                                          257
*Glossary*                                                          259

# Foreword

JON M. HUNTSMAN SR.

*The Huntsman Cancer Institute*

"Jon, you have cancer."

These words from my doctor, on an otherwise ordinary day in late 1991, hit me with almost unbearable force. Suddenly, I knew how it felt to have your blood run cold.

Like millions of other Americans who receive this diagnosis every year, I was stunned, anguished, and terrified—as if I had just received a guilty verdict for a crime I didn't commit.

I had been enjoying a healthy, active, productive life. At age 54, I was in my prime. My just-completed annual physical examination showed me to be in excellent health. But a happenstance drop-by at a local fitness center resulted in a doctor's taking a blood sample and running a PSA test. This test indicated the possibility of prostate cancer and it clearly saved my life, as subsequent biopsies confirmed that I had the disease.

There were so many things I still wanted to do, so much that I hoped to give. Although I had faced many obstacles during my life, I had always felt particularly blessed. I had a loving family and friends, a prosperous global business that provided jobs for thousands of people, and a true zest for life.

But now I had prostate cancer—the cancer that is most common among males and is second only to lung cancer as a killer of American men. I had always believed that things happen to us for a reason, that God has a plan for each of His children. I had great faith that this, too, would pass.

More than 200,000 men are diagnosed with prostate cancer each year in the United States, and 42,000 die from it. But thanks to early detection—which is the most critical aspect of survivability—I had time to amass the latest research data and to explore my treatment options fully before taking the next step. Prostate cancer survivor General Norman Schwarzkopf put it succinctly: "For me, it was like war. First thing you do is learn about the enemy."

I made a concerted effort to find doctors I trusted and respected—people who would work *with* me, not "for me" or "on me." I opened up to those closest to me and derived great strength from their love and prayers. I decided to face my cancer squarely, to fight it with all my might and, ultimately, to win.

My most valuable ally in this battle, as throughout our marriage, was my beloved wife, Karen. She was by my side, a radiant source of inner peace every step of the way.

In January 1992, I underwent five hours of surgery at the University of Utah Health Sciences Center for removal of my prostate gland. Subsequent pathology tests indicated the cancer had not spread to my lymph nodes or elsewhere, but the disease had totally encapsulated my prostate. The next six months were virtual torture.

My bout with cancer left me with greater strength and faith and with an intensified feeling of oneness with my fellow man. It also left me with a vision: I vowed to launch one of the country's preeminent cancer research institutes—a foundation devoted exclusively to helping eradicate the scourge of cancer—all cancers. This was not a fleeting impulse; it was and continues to be a deep passion. My mother died of breast cancer and my father was victimized by prostate cancer.

As one in five men will contract prostate cancer at some point in his life, research is imperative, and the need for funding for prostate cancer research is great. This disease is not the only one commonly referred to as a silent killer, but it is distinguished by the silence of its victims and potential victims. It is just now coming out of the closet, according to Dr. William Fair of the Memorial Sloan-Kettering Cancer Center in New York. Men have been reluctant to speak out about a disease that is so intensely personal with its haunting specter of impotence and incontinence. The National Cancer Institute spent $1.8 billion on breast cancer from 1990 to 1997 and only $376 million on prostate cancer. My goal, and the goal of the contributors to this book, is to help instigate sweeping studies that will benefit those afflicted with cancer in all its forms.

Thus in 1995, my family established the Huntsman Cancer Institute at the University of Utah with an initial contribution of $100 million and an additional $51 million we had raised. The Huntsman Cancer Institute is committed to discovering genetic and molecular solutions that will interrupt cancer development at its earliest stages and provide innovative therapies for later-stage cancers. We are in the process of building a team of world-renowned specialists from a variety of disciplines who will do their groundbreaking work from our seven-story, state-of-the-art building, scheduled for completion in late 1998, adjacent to the University of Utah Health Sciences Center.

In the meantime, cancer survivors have each other, which is a priceless resource. That community, in large part, is what this book is all about, and I am privileged to introduce it to you. Media coverage of prostate cancer has increased dramatically during the past few years, but up to now, it has been largely clinical, rarely exploring the pathos and poignancy behind the scenes. That's where this book comes in.

The stories of these remarkable men and women are supplemented with an exhaustive, up-to-date overview of prostate cancer, beginning with basic anatomy and encompassing detailed facts about testing, research, and the confusing array of treatment options. The book also provides a wonderfully well conceived, step-by-step instruction manual, even including daily schedule suggestions and nutrition-packed recipes that can help create a sense of order during this tumultuous time.

Most significant, however, are the messages of the ten prostate cancer survivors and four of their wives whose experiences make up this volume. These survivors have performed a profound act of generosity: They have become teachers in the finest sense of the word by selflessly giving to others the benefit of their experiences. They share their most wrenching and intimate emotions as well as the highly instructive details of their quests for renewed health. Their candid, moving accounts will empower you to cope with both the disease and with the overwhelming waves of conflicting emotions that could compromise your resolve. As their stories demonstrate, coping with the disease can be demeaning as well as terrifying if one is not informed. Solid data are the best weapons, emotionally as well as physiologically. This collection makes available to the reader an articulate, compassionate, and knowledgeable support group—a critical ally in any man's struggle. It keeps humanity, not cancer, at the forefront, and it could help recently diagnosed prostate cancer patients and their families to transform bitterness and rage into the life-affirming energy to convert a calamity into a challenge.

If you have prostate cancer, you *must* take charge. Being passive— lying back and waiting for the doctor to run the show—is a perilous strategy indeed. Ironically, the disease that many characterize as a threat to their manhood demands those very qualities traditionally associated with manhood: strength, courage, decisiveness, and dignity. All of the survivors profiled in this book emerged from their ordeal as better human beings. Several say they are happier and more fulfilled than ever before and that their good marriages got better. Their values and lifestyles were altered; their spirituality, humility, and feelings of love were enhanced. After cancer, they conclude, a man realizes what is really important.

Although the book reminds you that you are not alone—millions of men will confront prostate cancer—it also emphasizes that each patient is special and brings his own set of needs and strengths to the process. The book portrays the extraordinary reservoirs of character that the most "ordinary" people possess. Heroism and nobility repose in all of us, waiting to be employed. The battle, wrenching though it is, can also be a celebration of life.

Please know that my thoughts and prayers are with you.

## Notes

Jon Huntsman Sr. is chairman of the Huntsman Corporation, a bulk-chemical business based in Salt Lake City, Utah, and a prostate cancer survivor. He recently established the Huntsman Cancer Institute, where medical researchers are working to find a cure for cancer.

# Preface

PEGGY MCCARTHY

*President, McCarthy Medical Marketing*

In her book *Kitchen Table Wisdom*, Rachel Naomi Remen, M.D., states, "Everybody is a story." Prior to the takeover of our lives by television and, more recently, by corporate technology, people did sit around the kitchen table and tell stories. With the advent of television, much of that communication time among family members and friends was lost . . . at least until the launch of the Internet. But it is not only within groups of family and friends but between patient and physician that communication has been diminished. Managed care, of course, has severely diminished the time a physician actually can or will spend talking with and really listening to a patient. In managed care—and sadly, as in most of our lives—time is perceived as money, and few of us take time to sit around the examining table, the office desk, or the kitchen table and really communicate.

This book is based on the interactions of a group of ten men and some of their spouses who sat around a large table for four-and-a-half days telling their stories about living with prostate cancer. It is a book about strength and courage. It is also about trust, love, and friendship and about finding new life pathways not imagined before the diagnosis of prostate cancer. And it is about intense loss and grief and about the gifts that a diagnosis of cancer brings if we are open to those gifts. One of those gifts—for the men living with the diagnosis of prostate cancer and for their families and other loved ones and their health care providers—is the gift of honesty. The idea for this book derived from my colleagues and my desire to bring information not readily available to men diagnosed with prostate cancer and their loved ones, as well as to the health professionals who treat them. Over the years, as my colleagues and I have focused more and more on cancer education, we have developed a strong belief that informed decisionmaking by patients is imperative for healing to take place. Informed decisionmaking means that patients, their family members, and the health professionals who work with them throughout the disease process all work together—openly and honestly—as colleagues. We are grateful that Janssen Pharmaceutica recognized the need and the value of this book's messages and generously funded its development through an educational grant.

This book examines the lives of ten men and their families who have been living with prostate cancer. It is about their decisionmaking—some of which was based on solid information and some of which was based on the belief that decisions needed to be made very quickly and the physicians treating them knew best. But this book is mostly about ten men who have searched, have learned, have grown—in their belief in themselves as they research information and become more involved in decisionmaking; in their abilities to communicate with their loved ones and their compatriots who, like themselves, are living with prostate cancer; and in their willingness and desire to make their wishes known to their health providers and caregivers.

Living with prostate cancer is, for most men and their loved ones, a learning process full of challenges. The initial diagnosis often means dashed hopes and dreams. For everyone involved, it means soul-searching about the meaning of life and asking the question "Why me?" These men and their partners demonstrate the struggles that are faced in learning to cope with this disease and the treatments—and the side effects of both. They showed true courage by listening to and talking with total strangers about bodily functions that most men consider very private and that they may have, prior to their diagnosis, only joked about with locker-room humor. Few of us have the nerve to discuss such personal issues even with our physicians or loved ones—much less with a group of strangers sitting around a table in a retreat center—without blinking an eye.

Our society has, in the past, placed a mantle of responsibility on the medical community to be all-knowing and all-powerful. This expectation has changed in the past few years as more and more people are learning that they must actively participate in their own health care decisionmaking if they are to receive optimum treatment. This realization may be the most important effect of managed care for both patients and physicians.

Consumers have access, as never before, to a wide variety of medical information in books, on the Internet, on television, and in support groups. Fewer people are willing to turn complete responsibility for their health care and health care decisions over to their doctors. This change benefits doctors as well as patients. Physicians no longer are considered godlike in their wisdom and thus don't have to pretend to be infallible in their recommendations and decisions or to carry the weight of that image when the outcomes of those decisions are not favorable.

Because patients and their families are much more knowledgeable, they are much quicker to anger when a treatment causes more side effects than expected or when a therapy is not made available to them, especially if that therapy could produce better outcomes. Now, more than ever, it is crucial that health care professionals learn to communicate honestly and openly with patients and their families about the recommendations and to welcome their input. And they must learn to understand that their role is not just to treat but also to recognize and address quality-of-life issues. Health care professionals must be willing to sit down at a table with their patients to learn what is important to them through the entire disease trajectory, especially if the disease progresses and it is evident that prostate cancer will become the cause of death. This is the time when "kitchen table" talk is most important and, sadly, when it least often occurs.

Patients and families, too, need to learn to ask questions assertively, to state their needs openly and clearly, and to accept responsibility for being partners in the decisionmaking process. More open communication can build trust and respect. Of course, the hope is for a cure, and a cure is what every contributor to this book works for. For some, the cure may be a spiritual healing that allows them to understand the process of dying without anger and hostility. This healing can best take place when there is true trust and respect among all players in this most dramatic of life's experiences.

All of us involved in the development of this book thank this group of ten wonderful men and their spouses who were able to attend the retreat. We thank them for their honesty, their willingness to share their grief, sorrows, and joys, and their time. We have learned so much from each of them and greatly value the friendships that were forged around our table.

# Acknowledgments

I would like to thank the following people for their time, support, and contributions to this book: Bill Dehn and Murray Corwin, the Prostate Forum; the late Jim Mullen, Man to Man Inc.; the late Lloyd Ney, PAACT; Hank Porterfield, US TOO International, Inc.; Susan Swanson, Prostate Cancer Support Group, Legacy Cancer Services, Portland, Oregon; and the staff of McCarthy Medical Marketing (MMM), with a very special thanks to Jo An Loren, editor-in-chief, and Peggy McCarthy, president of MMM, without whose ideas, vision, and guidance this book would not have been possible.

*Nadine Jelsing*

# About the Contributors

It would be difficult to gather together ten more different men. We are of different ethnicities and personalities. We live in different parts of the country and are involved in or retired from totally different careers.

However, we do share one common bond. We have all faced the diagnosis of prostate cancer. But once again, our differences are apparent. Each of us reacted to the diagnosis uniquely, and each of us has taken our own personal approach to fighting this disease.

Perhaps curiosity was one of the reasons we each agreed to participate in this project. More important, we all had a strong desire to share experiences and help educate other men with this disease. With great anticipation, we took a chance of spending five days with nine strangers.

We think it was a chance well taken. What could have quickly dissipated into a meltdown of disagreements and uncomfortable politeness instead mushroomed into five days of mutual respect—and five days of free-flowing ideas and information. That, we believe, is what makes this book unique and worthwhile: ten men, ten philosophies, and ten uncensored approaches to living and dealing with this disease—at all levels.

Four of our wives also chose to come, and their participation makes this book very special, too. Several of the sessions were held jointly with them. In the others, we talked privately. Our wives also engaged in a private discussion session of their own.

We talked about everything. The sessions were loosely structured to make sure we incorporated issues important to everyone, such as diagnosis, treatment choices, side effects, and how our choices affected us, our partners, and our families. As the retreat progressed, however, many other topics spontaneously surfaced. Regardless of the subject matter, we tried to deal with each issue honestly and thoughtfully. We agreed and we disagreed. We laughed a lot and we cried, and we helped each other not just with passive support but by proactively offering our personal perspectives and suggestions for dealing with some of the difficult issues surrounding this disease.

Not content with the status quo, we also strategized for the future and discussed ways to catapult prostate cancer into the public eye. Ultimately, we bonded. There's no other way to say it.

All of our discussions were audiotaped. The transcripts of our conversations have been woven into narrative form, heavily laced with practical and scientific information. As you read this book, we hope that you feel as if you are part of our efforts, because you will be *listening* to many of our conversations just as they took place.

These are our personal stories and experiences. They add up to a lot of hindsight meant to help you as you gather your own information and make your own choices about what to do. Like each of us, you will need to find your own way and what works best for you.

We also came to the retreat to help educate the health care provider. We want you—the doctors and the nurses—to read this book, too. If you do, you'll find out what we need from you and how we wish to be treated; only by working together as partners can we optimize care. So please read the book with an open mind, realizing that our goal is to improve and maximize the doctor-patient relationship. The benefits will truly affect everyone.

Finally, we want readers with prostate cancer to know that we are not supermen. We are men just like you. We have faced the same dilemmas, fears, and insecurities and have been forced to make tough decisions. Yet we have persevered and moved forward. Each day we have become a little more knowledgeable and a little more confident in ourselves and our ability to choose what is right for us. And little by little, we have become empowered. Empowerment is, perhaps, what being a survivor is all about.

Before we begin, we want you to know a little bit about us and how we spend a *typical* day. We wrote these brief narratives personally, so what follows is an intimate glimpse into each of our lives.

**Paul Georgeades:** I am 63 years old and live with my wife, Phyllis, in Vancouver, Washington. We have three sons and eight grandchildren. I was diagnosed with Stage D1 prostate cancer in 1992 at 59 years of age.

I am a retired construction electrician. Over the years, I've traveled the country to work on a variety of industrial and commercial construction projects. Some of those projects have included the Twin Towers in New York City and the Golden Gate Bridge in San Francisco. I've also worked as an estimator for large construction jobs, and I held the position of electrical inspector for the city of Portland, Oregon in the 1970s.

Besides the fact that I got paid very well for these jobs, I also enjoyed that I was challenged mentally by each new job and, by the sheer nature of construction work, challenged physically, too. Each new job also brought the opportunity to meet many interesting people.

Although my construction days may be behind me, Phyllis and I still manage several rental properties in the area. We also try to devote a good portion of our time to doing things that really make us happy. Traveling is one of them. I love to travel everywhere and anywhere, and I've managed to tie that in with another hobby of mine, which is rock collecting. I've found samples of beautiful rocks from all over the United States, including specimens of obsidian, emerald, and sapphire. Back home, you'll often find me at my computer. I'm still learning how to use it.

Like most people, I find it hard to pinpoint a typical day, but I usually start mine by fixing Phyllis and myself a cup of tea. Then we plan the rest of the day. Foremost we try to do something together daily, whether shopping or taking a drive together. There's always yardwork to do and odds and ends around the house that need my attention. We have long-standing jobs as baby-sitters for our grandkids. We just can't seem to get fired no matter what we do! All kidding aside, our three sons and the eight grandchildren are the joy of our lives, and spending time with and enjoying our family is at the top of our list of things that please.

Speaking of family, I've been having fun tracing my roots and have come up with some interesting characters—including a great-grandfather from Ireland who fought in the Civil War and some colorful Greek sculptors. Music has also captured my attention. I recently bought an old piano at an auction, took it apart, cleaned, polished, and repaired it, and put it back together—and it works. Now I'm trying to teach myself to play it. It's something new. It's another challenge and I thrive on challenges.

I've noticed one bad "side effect" of getting older. It's that I seem to be getting slower and slower, but the days are going by faster and faster. For me, the days seem to slip by much too quickly, and I feel that I won't be able to accomplish all that I want to in life. This is something I have no control over, and such things frustrate me—kind of like the IRS.

I feel that I was very fortunate to have been diagnosed when I was. My wife deserves my appreciation and a lot of the credit for my being alive today, as do all my doctors, the medicines, and the treatments. All elements combined have given me six years of survivorship. I feel that I owe a lot of people a lot of thanks.

I want all men to know the importance of early detection. If you're 40 years old or over, get tested. Go *before* you begin having any symptoms. Have that digital rectal exam (DRE) or that PSA test NOW! They don't hurt, they're easy, and they may save your life.

**Aarol (Bud) Irish:** I am 74 years old. My wife, Elaine, and I are fortunate to have two places to call home. During the summer we live in Saginaw, Michigan, and in the winter months we head to Venice, Florida. We have been married for 51 years and have ten children—five sons and five daughters. I was diagnosed originally with Stage B2 prostate cancer in December 1989 at age 67. In January 1990, further testing revealed Stage C2 or possibly D1 cancer.

I'm retired and was a general agent for Union Mutual Insurance Company for 35 years. I was involved primarily in life insurance, disability, and the pension business. I think the most satisfaction came from planning good life insurance plans for friends and clients, plans that in many cases provided funds for their children's education. In the event of some deaths, life insurance kept families together and saved businesses, and I felt pretty good about that.

I also feel good about working with my wife in raising and educating our family. Elaine managed the house, I managed four businesses, and together we managed the family. In the early family years, I was a Boy Scout leader and a YMCA grade school basketball coach. I have taken a great deal of pride in watching my children go through high school and college and head out into the world with good occupations.

I've always been very civic minded. I sat on the board of the Saginaw Chamber of Commerce, was president of our local Lions Club,

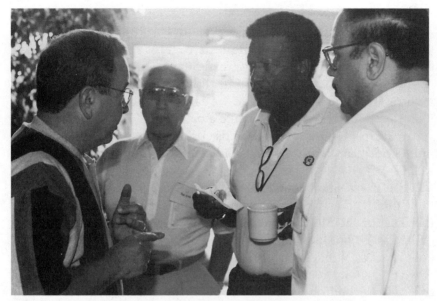

Manuel Vazquez, Bud Irish, Bob White, Virgil Simons

and was state president of the Michigan Association of Life Under-writers, followed by six years as the national committee man. I am also a life member of the VFW. In 1965, I also started giving speeches on positive thinking.

For me there's no such thing as a dull day, and I always manage to have plenty to do. I start early, about 7:30 A.M. At least two mornings a week, Elaine and I go to mass and communion. I love playing tennis, and I try to play several times a week—both recreational and tournament. Music is another love. I learned to play the guitar as a boy and haven't stopped for the past 65 years.

I get plenty of mail and usually try to spend an hour or two daily in correspondence. Since 1989, I've made it my business to study and research treatments for prostate cancer and have given dozens of speeches and answered thousands of phone calls. I talk with people from all over the country who are newly diagnosed with the disease or who are doing well and living normal lives after treatment. Closer to home, I have breakfast meetings or coffee with prostate cancer patients two or three times a week. I've also been very active in the support groups Man to Man and PAACT.

Working outdoors is also a great love of mine. We own 179 acres of woods in Michigan. It's been very enjoyable for me to spend time preserving and clearing some of the acreage. My wife and I also like to travel and visit our families spread out across the country.

My philosophy has been "In all things always do your best and then in God you leave the rest." That seems to prevent me from worrying lots of times after I make a decision.

I treasure my family and friends. I find that the older I get, the more I find that family, friends, and memories are the greatest things in life.

When I was small I remember sitting at my parents' dining room table and reading two hand-painted framed verses that hung on either side of the old-fashioned sideboard. These verses made an indelible mark on my life: "It's easy enough to be pleasant when life goes by like a song, but the man worthwhile is the one with a smile when everything goes dead wrong" and "Never say die; up man and try." The second one was very special to me during World War II when I spent 43 months with the 102nd Mechanized Calvary Reconnaisance throughout Europe.

I feel life should have a purpose, and in later life I've learned that people without a purpose are like a kite without wind: It's difficult to get anywhere. For me, advocating for prostate cancer awareness is one of the most important and worthwhile things I can do. I will continue to give talks to groups across the United States, and I will continue to respond to phone calls and inquiries from prostate cancer patients. I feel the greatest thing I can do is give these people peace of mind and tell them that today there are wonderful doctors, drugs, and, depending on their belief, a wonderful God. Combine all this with a little good luck, prayers, and the many ways of combating this disease and I think it helps eliminate much of the fear and stress.

As for me, I am not afraid to die but have a great desire to live.

**John Plosnich:** I am 72 years old and live with my wife, Rosalie, in Oak Brook, Illinois. I was diagnosed with Stage B1 prostate cancer in 1991 at age 67.

I am retired from my business, Plosnich & Associates, which manufactures machine tools. The field of technology has always fascinated me, and I am well aware of the scientific potential and brainpower that's out there. We just have to harness some of that power and put it to work in prostate cancer research. I also served in the U.S. Navy during World War II.

My life continues to be active, happy, and fulfilling. I am one of the directors of the support group US TOO International in Hinsdale, Illinois. Much of my time is spent on the phone counseling the thousands of newly diagnosed patients who call our offices looking for information, hope, and support. I remember with intense clarity what I went through as a result of my own ignorance of this disease, and I wish that on no one. I'm very proud of having received US TOO's highest Eagle Award for Survivorship in 1993.

My days are always filled from top to bottom. An ongoing project of my wife's and mine is the renovation of our home. We were flooded several years ago, and we've still got boxes to unpack and much work to do. But no matter how busy I am, one thing I never forgo is daily exercise. I hit the treadmill every day and try to log about three miles daily. Sometimes I'll incline it in order to work up a real sweat. If you're a cancer patient, it's important to try to exercise a little bit each day. That goes double for me because I'm also a heart patient. I feel that I'm exercising my mind, body, and spirit all at once.

I have a strong appreciation for the great outdoors and enjoy golf, fishing, and other outdoor activities. Rosalie and I love the natural beauty and satisfaction we find in a simple walk together outside. In fact, we are a team in every way and cherish the gift of our companionship. We dine together often at the country club we belong to and also find great joy cultivating our many friendships. I try to reserve regular lunch dates with old friends, and Rosalie and I like to take in a movie and dinner with friends once a week. We're also involved with a local theater group and enjoy the arts, music, and world travel. I am a firm believer in living one day at a time, having fun, and sharing that fun with family and friends.

One of our most pressing goals is to try to help promising researchers with their work in prostate cancer, and Rosalie and I are busy setting up various foundations and trusts to ensure funding. We must find a cure for this disease. Many treatments, including mine, are only temporary. We need a cure, and I will continue to fight for more recognition and more research money until one is found.

We also need to get information about this disease out to men and their families, and we need to get out the message of hope. Men and their families need to know that although facing this disease will be a challenge, a diagnosis is not the end of the world.

If, in any way, my advocacy work furthers the fight against prostate cancer, I'll feel that all my efforts have been worthwhile.

**Charlie Russ:** I am 70 years old and live with my wife, Marcia, in Leawood, Kansas, a suburb of greater Kansas City. We have five children. I was diagnosed with prostate cancer (stage unknown at diagnosis, but currently D2) in 1991 at age 65.

I have held senior positions in law and human resources, including corporate assistant labor relations director and field personnel director of Montgomery Ward; assistant state's attorney, Cook County, Illinois; and vice president of Personnel and Labor Relations for a $400 million Midwest company.

I'm happy that I was commissioned an infantry officer in World War II at age 19, that I graduated from Notre Dame magna cum laude, that I received my J.D. from the University of Chicago, and that I was elected to the *Law Review*.

My greatest achievement is my family. Marcia is a great wife. Lisa, Jane, and Nina are bright, successful, and beautiful daughters, and Jane has our four wonderful grandchildren. Charlie III and Benjamin are all that you could ever ask of your sons in any way.

Working as an assistant state's attorney served my Type A, overachiever personality well. I got a great deal of satisfaction working as a trial lawyer and putting away a lot of "bad guys." I also find satisfaction being involved in neighborhood and civic issues and have been an officer and board member of numerous organizations in Chicago, Detroit, and Kansas City, including Rotary International and the Salvation Army. I've also published many articles on the subject of human resources and other subjects.

I founded and currently run my own human resources consulting business (Charles Russ Associates), which helps companies solve people problems. We help them hire and promote more qualified people; reduce turnover; intensify customer service; raise trust levels; and improve connections, teamwork, relationships, and commitment. I love it.

A typical day for me starts around 7:30 A.M. with exercise on a stationary bicycle. Then I shower and have breakfast, which always includes plenty of fresh fruit. Oftentimes I'll have lunch with my wife at the local hospital, where she works as a medical technologist, or with friends or clients.

A great deal of my time is spent as chairman of LAC-PAACT, the Legal Action Committee of Patient Advocates for Advanced Prostate Cancer (PAACT), a 33,000-member patient advocate organization. We have been very successful in having judges review patient coverage denials under Medicare, especially in cases involving cryotherapy. In fact, through much hard work and persistence, I persuaded the American Urological Association (AUA) to recognize cryotherapy as being no longer experimental or investigational.

Recently, I've also been appointed the fund-raising chairman of PAACT and its liaison to US TOO International. So you can see I spend many, many hours a week dealing with our lawyers and acting as a national support person to dozens of member patients all over the country who contact me for advice. This type of advocacy work for prostate cancer survivors and their families is very important to me. It's vital that we keep fighting for our rights as cancer patients and our right to know about and have access to all treatment options, as well as preserve the doctor-patient relationship, which I believe is being destroyed by Medicare and the Washington bureaucracy.

More often than not, you'll find me at my computer in my home office, typing and strategizing on the phone at the same time. It seems as if there is not enough time in the day to accomplish all I want to do in life, and I often work seven days a week trying.

What frustrates me most is seeing uninformed patients making uninformed decisions about their health. Patients need to empower themselves by learning as much about prostate cancer as they can before they start making decisions that will affect their lives forever. They need to become equal partners with their doctors. PAACT did this for me.

I do find time to relax, and I'm trying to cut back on work to make more time to relax. That's been tough because I'm the type of person who likes to be involved up to my eyeballs in projects. I hope to do more traveling, which I've already started doing, and I've also recently discovered mystery novels and reading again.

I enjoy solving problems and keeping up with friends and classmates from the University of Chicago, for which I write a column on UC class activities. I regularly write columns for the PAACT newsletter as well.

I also enjoy spending time with my family and keep in close touch with my children on a weekly basis. Playing the piano is also a much-loved pastime. In fact, you'll find a Steinway grand taking center stage in my living room. Another big part of the family culture revolves around the University of Notre Dame. As an ex-cheerleader, I attend football games every year, and we also have a family burial plot there. It's a sacred place to me.

Although I have had strong differences, legal and professional, with the medical profession, I continue to use the best that traditional medicine has to offer, combined with alternative therapies, and I try to maintain a positive mental outlook. I have a strong faith in God and a strong support team that has helped me through some stressful times.

If there is one word that would describe why I came to this gathering, it's empowerment. That means taking the time to understand this disease, taking charge of your health care, making informed choices and better choices, and fighting for better solutions. It also means fighting for what you believe is right for you and for others.

**Virgil Simons:** I am 50 years old and live with my wife, Jennifer, and two dogs in Secaucus, New Jersey. I was diagnosed with Stage B2 prostate cancer in 1995 at age 49.

I am a textile sales executive. I develop new business for U.S. Knitting Mills and develop opportunities for selling fabrics to apparel manufacturers and industrial-military contractors. Getting new orders gives me a great deal of satisfaction, as does building working relationships with clients. I am a Vietnam veteran.

I'm usually up by 5:00 A.M. to feed, walk, and play with the dogs. Then I fix breakfast for Jennifer and myself, read the paper, and leave for work by 7:30. During the day you'll find me attending meetings, going out on calls, and handling the details of business.

I use my lunch hour to work on my prostate cancer advocacy programs to support other survivors and the newly diagnosed. There's e-mail to send and answer, a website to maintain, and other writing to do. After dinner at home with my wife, I usually pick up my advocacy work again: correspondence, mailing out proposals, preparing brochures, and developing new vehicles to advance the cause. Sometimes I don't stop until midnight or later.

My life has changed dramatically since my diagnosis. When I was 48 I was fit, active, healthy, and enjoying the pleasures of life and just coming of age with a new sense of self-awareness, acceptance, and future hopes. Then came my diagnosis and my introduction to the beast. I felt anger at an unfair God and cursed the fates that had dealt more than my share of troubles. I found myself letting self-pity wash over me and fighting the fear of cancer, which was consuming my life and tormenting me day and night. Finally I said, "Drive on!!!" I was going to live, on my terms and not cancer's.

I quickly realized that I didn't know what I didn't know. Doctors could not be totally relied on because their recommendations often had the bias of their training, disciplines, and peers; nor could friends, who could offer only thirdhand experience or tell me what worked for them. I found out that I needed to know as much about this new world as possible and ultimately discovered that the computer and the Internet provided answers. They were tangible weapons against an intangible beast. I found the power to explore the choices of weapons available for the battle and the power to say, "This is *my* life and I will live it as I choose."

As I went through the whole process prior to my surgery and recovery, I met and talked with many people who were also lost in choices or the results of the choices they had made or that had been made for them. Often their anguish was palpable, their dreams diminished, and hope all but gone—all because they didn't have the power. The insidious thing about cancer is that it not only robs you of your health and maybe your life, it affects your partner and sometimes [their] perception of you, it affects your family, and it affects your finances; and it can ultimately destroy dreams. Thus was my baptism into becoming an advocate for change. I was determined to give new meaning to the phrase "Power to the People!!"

I've found a new purpose in life that goes beyond just the monetary (although I'm still far from becoming a socialist—Dom Perignon and I are ace boon buddies!), and I've found a new satisfaction and contentment in my life. All of the dreams for career and utilization of the skills I possess as an executive are coming together in my new role as an advocate at the same time that I am doing well. A life force surges inside that I haven't felt ever before, and I want to ride the crest. I love walking down a street on a sunny day and picking up the energy around me, spending time with my family, tennis, movies, theater, and travel.

What frustrates me is dealing with "mental midgets"—people who can't see past their own parochial issues—and having to compromise personal principles for business expediency. I also hate not being able to use all my abilities on a regular business basis.

I don't know what lies ahead of me from a health standpoint. But in actuality, I don't think about the beast on a daily basis. I refuse to let it have any dominance over me, my life, or my dreams. If the cancer returns, I'll deal with it then, but until and unless it returns, it doesn't exist. Only the work is important: to help others and to take the battle to the next level—and me along with it.

**Peter Stults:** I am 65 years old and live with my wife, Cindy, and our 15-year-old son in Sarasota, Florida. I have three other children from a prior marriage. I was diagnosed with Stage C prostate cancer in 1990 at age 59.

I spent my first 20 years after graduation with Eastman Kodak and Booz Allen & Hamilton, management consultants, in administrative and financial management. My last position was as administrative vice president for three of the Booz Allen companies. During this period of my life, I pretty much kept my nose to the grindstone and I fared well. My primary strength was in being able to keep "six balls up in the air at one time," as the president of the company once said.

The past 20 years were spent building my own businesses here in Florida: an insurance premium finance company, a boat-chartering business, an executive suite (two locations), and a temporary help service (T.O.P.S. Personnel) with five offices in southwest Florida.

With my own small companies, I was much more aggressive and creative. After I got them pretty well established (so I wasn't worrying about where my next meal was coming from), I sort of played with business. In other words, I didn't keep my nose to the grindstone. I was divorced during this time, and so I owned and lived on a decommissioned 93-foot Canadian Navy submarine detection vessel and played weekend sailor with my friends, up and down the west coast of Florida, for five years before remarrying and settling back into a somewhat more conventional lifestyle.

Until my retirement, shortly after I was diagnosed with prostate cancer, I kept two or three companies going at once, and I had a lot of fun making innovative changes in the way each of the businesses operated. I have now disposed of all the businesses except T.O.P.S. Personnel, which my wife currently runs. (I'm still chairman of the board.)

I enjoyed being successful!!! When my businesses were doing well, I felt great and on top of the world. When they were struggling, I would have aches and pains and couldn't sleep. We have been fortunate that our businesses did well most of the time.

Now that I'm retired, my life is filled with doing BIG THINGS . . . and little things. I'm president of Man to Man Inc., in Sarasota, Florida . . . and I'm the taxi for our 15-year-old son around town. I'm active in school PTA-type functions . . . and clean up the messes of our dog and two cats. I handle our investments . . . and do the food shopping. I'm heavily involved in real estate investing and rehabilitation . . . and do roughly half the dishes and laundry. I'm the district director of the National Prostate Cancer Coalition . . . and do most of the cooking.

I also handle frequent referral calls from Sarasota Memorial Hospital and the local American Cancer Society office, counseling mostly newly diagnosed prostate cancer patients. So as you can see, my current "portfolio" is a mixed bag.

Being successful isn't the only thing that makes me happy. I like feeling healthy; being busy; finding my family happy with their lives; listening to music; seeing a sunrise or sunset or the stars on a black, black night. I love being enveloped by the scent of jasmine, gardenias, or other sweet-smelling flowering plants and seeing the alligators, turtles, anhingas, and great blue herons in the pond on one of our properties.

I hate seeing people hurt or unhappy and cruelty to living things. And it is sometimes difficult for me to deal with my periodic bouts of bad health (I also deal with diabetes, hypertension, and rheumatoid arthritis) and my impotence from my treatments for prostate cancer. I also hate inefficiency, bureaucratic bumbling, and focusing on minor, unimportant details in life.

All said and done, I'd like to be seen as someone who cares about people, is continuing to become more knowledgeable about my disease, and is available to provide whatever support I can as the newly diagnosed enter into this unasked-for path that is now before them. It's important for the newly diagnosed patient to know that I was dumber than dumb about prostate cancer before my diagnosis. I couldn't even spell the word. But I have learned a lot, and I think it's important for all prostate cancer patients to be knowledgeable because, ultimately, they have to make the final treatment decisions.

I'd also like them to know that prostate cancer doesn't necessarily have to "ruin" their lives. I'd much rather not have the disease, but I feel good about myself and life, and I'd sure rather be where I am now than six feet under. I've learned that human beings can be very flexible and resourceful, and by and large I've adjusted to my changed condition.

Having to face my mortality when I was sailing blithely and blindly along was definitely a shock—a big shock. But that's part of growing up, too. Right now, I'm enjoying being alive.

**Manuel Vazquez:** I am 57 years old and live with my wife, Mary, in Houston, Texas. This is a second marriage for both of us. Mary has two daughters from her first marriage, and I had six children from mine—four sons and two daughters. I was diagnosed with Stage B2 prostate cancer in 1994 at age 55.

For nearly 30 years I worked in the Information Technology Department of a large oil company. Most of those years were spent in mainframe computer operations and seven were in administration, which included large-scale computer leasing, software administration, and asset management. I also developed a collection system for the recovery of outstanding accounts receivable and trained new personnel in computer operations. I loved my job and the fact that I was on the cutting edge of a revolutionary technology.

I came to the United States from Cuba, with my first wife, as a refugee from communism. My first son was born some 40 hours after we arrived in this country. I was 23 years old, literally penniless, and couldn't speak a word of English.

Unfortunately, I was downsized from the oil company a year ago, but that opened up a whole new opportunity for me. I was too young to retire, so I embarked on a new career in the same field of computer operations at the help desk of the Houston Police Department. I have come to love this job as well, and I feel very useful as a civil servant for the city.

A typical day for me is extremely busy. I have a wide range of interests and hobbies outside of work. These interests include world history, sociology, reading, and listening to classical music. At times, I get virtually glued to my computer surfing the Internet (my wife is a self-professed Internet widow). On weekends we like to garden together, entertain, and cook very low-fat gourmet dishes with lots of fruits and vegetables. I have to admit that prior to my diagnosis, I did not have very good eating habits. My wife and I restored the house we're presently living in from the ground up, and that endeavor has made us very proud of all of our hard work. If I can find some spare time, I'm hoping to further express myself artistically by creating mosaics with tile, and with pottery.

I am a ten-year volunteer at Omega House (an AIDS hospice) doing primary patient care. I think I've gotten a lot more out of it than I've put into it. Working at the hospice, I've learned to deal with death and dying, and that has helped prepare me for my own death—which I don't plan to experience any time soon.

Overall, I think of myself as a happy person. However, being sexually impotent from my treatment for prostate cancer is very frustrating and causes me a great deal of distress. I do realize, though, that I have traded my sexuality for my life. After all, there's no sex at all six feet under. I choose life.

I am also a member of the board of the Tex Us Too prostate cancer support group (the largest in Houston) and am active in prostate cancer interest groups on the Internet. In fact, the activity that brings me the most satisfaction is reaching out to fellow prostate cancer patients when they are newly diagnosed. My goal is to bring them out of silent despair into hope by giving them information and support.

Another way I do this is by working regularly with the American Cancer Society's Man to Man Visitation Program. This is a pilot program designed after the very successful Reach to Recovery Program for women with breast cancer. So far, we're not getting as many referrals from doctors as we would like to have, but we realize that it took women survivors 25 years to get to where they are now—reaching their breast cancer sisters. I am also a member of the American Cancer Society Speaker's Bureau, spreading the gospel of early detection at churches, wellness programs, and so on, and I have participated in Spanish-language radio programs to make people aware of the disease.

Coming home from work each day, I usually have a message from someone newly diagnosed with prostate cancer or someone I need to follow up on. I have gotten calls from all over and once had the opportunity to serve a patient who came to Houston all the way from New Zealand for surgery. We are fortunate to have an outstanding medical center in Houston.

In fact, hardly a week goes by without my having a new person to reach out to who has been newly diagnosed with prostate cancer.

Not only does this work continue to give me a great deal of personal satisfaction but it helps me cope with my own frustrations as well.

In reaching out to others I have come to this conclusion about my personal philosophy, and I quote from *In Search of Beyond*: "Let us keep this truth before us. You say you have no faith? Love—and faith will come. You say you are sad? Love—and joy will come. You say you are alone? Love—and you will break out of solitude. You say you are in hell? Love—and you will find yourself in heaven. Heaven is love."

Life is good!

**Bob White:** I am 66 years old and live with my wife, Sandy, in Westminster, California. We have five children and six grandchildren. I was diagnosed with Stage B1 prostate cancer in 1993 at age 63.

I spent 21 years as a Los Angeles police officer. My satisfaction from this job came primarily from working with youth, specifically the preteen kids. I tried to expose them to a different and better lifestyle within the police department's youth program, called Explorers.

I retired from the force in 1994 after being diagnosed with prostate cancer. Needless to say, without any knowledge of prostate cancer, I felt I would soon be retiring from life itself. I was scared and filled with denial.

My life had been relatively full to this point. Before joining the police department, I was, strangely enough, making a living as a professional entertainer; I sang and traveled with the Platters vocal group for ten years. My spare time was spent studying art. Music and art are still an integral part of my everyday life.

Now that I'm retired, it seems that my life is busier and more fulfilling than ever before. An average day begins for me with 20 to 30 minutes of meditation and reading spiritual material. I go regularly to a nearby park, where I walk a minimum of four miles a day. Later I go to the art studio where I paint and teach beginning drawing to children and adults three days a week.

I have also taken up studying the guitar, and I'm taking a computer class. All this keeps me quite busy.

Since my prostate cancer diagnosis, I have learned to value life—every minute, every hour, every day. I feel very blessed to still be around and enjoy a quality-filled life. I have altered my lifestyle to include eating better, exercising, and stopping to give thanks for my blessings. Cancer has humbled me.

I joined a local prostate cancer support group, which I found to be so instrumental in providing me the knowledge I have obtained about this disease. I serve on the board of directors and take every opportunity to help other men who have been diagnosed with the disease and are not informed about it.

I chose to participate in this book retreat with nine other men, whom I'd never met, mainly because I saw it as an opportunity to further the knowledge about prostate cancer; to maybe say or share something in print that may get through to one man with the disease who may feel as alone and helpless as I did at one time. If my contribution can benefit one individual, then my time and effort spent on helping produce this book will have been worthwhile.

I strongly urge all men 40 years of age and over to have a PSA test and a digital rectal exam (DRE). It could save your life. I especially urge African American men to have these tests because statistics state that one in nine is diagnosed with the disease as compared to one in eleven in other ethnicities.

Last, I have learned that prostate cancer does not have to be a death sentence.

**Derek Workman:** I am 66 years old. I have three children living in different locations in the United States and four grandchildren. I spend my summers in New Mexico and my winters on the Gulf of Mexico in Florida. I was diagnosed with Stage B2 prostate cancer in 1992 at age 62.

I am a retired U.S. Air Force fighter weapons controller. My responsibilities were many and included controlling U.S. and allied fighter aircraft en route to targets that we assigned to them for engagement on combat and training missions. I also controlled other aircraft on rescue, reconnaissance, and surveillance (spy) missions and monitored and upgraded the capabilities and reliability of radar equipment and the combat capabilities of air defense units. The job also included writing operational plans and procedures and training other officers to become combat ready as controllers.

Of all my responsibilities, the one that probably gave me the most satisfaction was controlling the fighters and knowing that I had destroyed more targets than anyone else when the numbers were tallied at the end of the mission.

My day usually starts about 7:00 A.M. Depending on where I'm living at the time, I go for a walk on the beach or a ride on my bike. Being retired, I enjoy the fact that I'm free to do pretty much as I please, when I please. I can do a little yardwork, if that's needed, or I can play golf or go fishing, which I try to do several days a week. One of my great loves is traveling. My significant other and I enjoy our leisurely trips back and forth between Florida and New Mexico. We get off the interstate and use the back roads to visit out-of-the-way spots and historical attractions. We also enjoy planning and going on shorter trips to see the sites in the state we're living in at the time.

I feel my biggest job right now is to advise other prostate cancer patients on how to become survivors—to help reduce their fears and frustrations and those of their families. I tell them to immediately get in touch with a support group that is run by patients and survivors, to read books and gather information that will help them emotionally, and to get a good urologist—and by that I mean one who is knowledgeable, competent, compassionate, and oriented toward successful patient care, not dollars. I also go with newly diagnosed patients to visit their doctors if they are uncomfortable talking to doctors. I need to ensure that those patients get the answers they need about treatment options and side effects. I also tell them to look at all the procedures that are available both locally and in other areas and to talk to other survivors who have been in a similar situation.

I am very active in support groups, and I get totally frustrated when I hear how poorly some medical professionals have treated many of the people I come in contact with. That is inexcusable. I tell patients to take a "report card" with them when they visit their doctor. That way they can make sure they ask pertinent questions, record the information, and write down any other thoughts or impressions they may have. I also tell patients to always get a second and even a third or fourth opinion if they feel that they need to. In most situations they have plenty of time to make up their minds.

My philosophy is that every man in the position of being diagnosed with prostate cancer is entitled to understand the full range of treatments available. With that understanding, he will be empowered to make the most intelligent decisions for himself.

What a man firmly believes is his best course of action. It will serve him best and represents the best opportunity for him to become a survivor.

**Don Zank:** I am 60 years old and live with my wife, Lynne, in Cedar Springs, Michigan. We have three children. I was diagnosed with Stage D prostate cancer in 1993 at age 57.

I am a farrier. I shoe horses. Most of my life I have worked around animals, which has given me a lot of personal satisfaction and happiness. Over the years, I've also learned a great deal from them—how they function, what makes them sick, what makes them well. A lot of what I've learned I've applied to my own health and well-being.

I make use of a lot of alternative therapies. Many of them are based on what I've learned in the animal world and complemented by recommendations from my biochemist, who keeps close tabs on what my body needs nutritionally. You'll learn more about all this later in the book, but as you'll see in this overview, alternative therapies are a big part of my life.

I'm usually up by 7:00 in the morning. The first thing on my agenda is preparing my morning supply of hot lemonade, which I make with distilled water (I drink only distilled water), maple syrup, hydrogen peroxide, and cayenne pepper. I try to drink the entire batch by noon. Next, I measure out the rest of my day's supply of water, to which I add 35 percent hydrogen peroxide. I also get out my day's supply of supplements for all three meals. Fruit is a big item on my daily menu, so I load a day's supply into my lunch box. I'm on the road a lot with my business, so I've got to leave the house well prepared with exactly what I need to eat and drink during the day. It's a pretty strict regimen, but routine breeds familiarity and comfort, and I'm used to it.

All of our animals need their breakfasts, too, so before I leave, I feed our two horses, cats, and one dog. After the chores are done, I usually try to head to the local coffee shop for a little personal time with a plain biscuit, coffee, and the morning paper.

Then it's off on my rounds of shoeing and trimming horses. I have a lot of people who depend on me, and I'm often booked for months in advance. Some of my clients are as far as 50 miles away from my home. Shoeing horses is hard work, but I enjoy working outdoors, being with the animals, and talking with the owners. In fact, it makes me very unhappy if I don't feel well enough to get up and go to work each morning.

After I've returned home, my work isn't quite finished. We have a wood-burning furnace that heats our home, so in the wintertime there's usually wood to be chopped for the evening and morning hours. Finally, I need to make sure I have all the supplies I'll need for the next day and that they're ready to go in the back of my truck.

I'm finally ready for a vegetarian dinner and maybe a little TV or even a ball game. I also enjoy hunting trips during the fall. I bow hunt, and I do eat venison.

I think of myself as a very strong-willed person. I know what I want and that includes making decisions based on what I know in the animal world. I can also be an impatient person. Waiting makes me unhappy. But then so do taxes and, if you haven't already guessed, sometimes the medical profession. I have used traditional medicine and it has served me well, but sometimes trying to work with medical professionals and deal with their attitude toward complementary therapies has been frustrating at best.

Satisfaction for me also comes from helping other men with prostate cancer. I talk with people from all over the country—I'm not sure how they get my number—and explain to them that they have to be informed of their options. I've found what works best for me. It may not be for everyone, but at least each caller will know what I'm all about before he hangs up—and that someone cares. Then, he can make up his own mind.

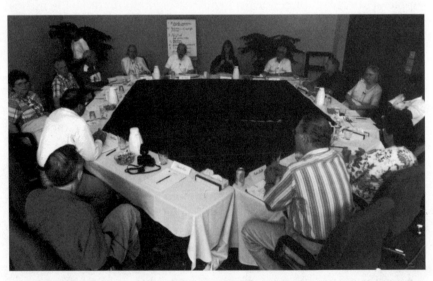

*Clockwise from poster:* John Plosnich, Nadine Jelsing, Bud Irish, Paul Georgeades, Phyllis Georgeades, Bob White, Mary Vazquez, Peter Stults, Charlie Russ, Virgil Simons, Lynne Zank, Don Zank, Derek Workman, Rosalie Plosnich

# 1

# *Diagnosis*

## A CHANGE IN PRIORITIES

*I've got prostate cancer. We all do, so let's see what we can do to encourage other people that the world has not come to an end.*
—*John Plosnich*

There are few people today who have not been touched by cancer. Maybe your mother had the disease—or your spouse or perhaps your grandfather or a friend. Intellectually, we all know that this disease exists, that it can strike randomly and unmercifully; but emotionally, we often feel that "it can never happen to *me*."

You have probably just found out otherwise and are now coming to grips with a life-altering proclamation: Your doctor has told you that you—yes *you*—have prostate cancer. Take a deep breath, because you immediately have two choices: You can ignore the situation and refuse to learn anything about it or you can start preparing yourself for the fight of your life. If you choose the latter, you're not alone. In fact, just by picking up this book, you have ten battle-seasoned warriors on your side.

We are ten men living with prostate cancer. We are men just like you with families, businesses, and responsibilities. But the fact that we have cancer has changed our lives. Some of those changes have been bad. Some of them have been good. In many ways, we think we've emerged as better men.

Our experiences, and all of them are as different as we are, have a common theme. We all knew virtually nothing about prostate cancer when we started this journey. That's not unusual, but as we quickly found out, it is dangerous. Dangerous because having prostate cancer entails making decisions, and ignorance can turn the

1

process into a game of Russian roulette with the highest of stakes: your health and, ultimately, your life. That's why we came together at this retreat: to share our stories with you, to spark your quest for knowledge, and to offer hope. Above all—to offer hope.

## The Dilemma

We consider ourselves to be strong men, both personally and professionally. We are successful in our respective careers, and we are used to taking charge and making decisions. Yet nothing we had done or learned prepared us for a diagnosis of prostate cancer. It came when we least expected it, and for some of us, it produced shock waves that challenged us to confront our own mortality, rocked our self-esteem, and jolted our conceptions of manhood.

"I was just staggered by it," recalled Peter, who got his diagnosis over the phone. "I knew nothing about it other than cancer—you die."

"All my thinking suddenly became very short term," said Paul. "When I went to buy toothpaste, I always got the small one. I didn't look for any green bananas. I remember thinking that I shouldn't upgrade my computer. There was no sense in that because I probably wouldn't be around to learn how to operate it."

When cancer struck us, it also struck those close to us. The diagnosis affected our partners as dramatically as it affected us. Bob remembers what it was like telling his wife. "We cried. We lay in bed and we cried. That was the first thing. Because we were ignorant. We knew nothing about this disease."

And Derek remembers wrestling with thoughts of inadequacy. "I was with a lady I had met 30 years ago and we had just gotten together again. And now I had cancer! I left her. It hurt me, it hurt her, and I felt very bad about it, but I also had the feeling that, well, I have prostate cancer, and I'm going to be impotent. At the time, I felt that's no life for me to present to her."

Don summed up what many of us felt: "When they hit you with this, it's devastating."

Devastating, staggering, you die. All strong images provoked by one word—cancer. Not all of us, however, started writing our obituaries. Some of us took a completely different view of the diagnosis—that of invincibility. For Bud, it stemmed from living through the horrors of World War II. "I had some experiences early in life that caused me to have no fear of death," he says. "In World War II, I spent 43 months in a mechanized cavalry reconnaissance troop, and a month before the war was over, I almost didn't come home. I was in a six-man patrol in Germany. We had four of our buddies killed. I was one of the ones left for dead. So when the doctor gave me the diagnosis, I tapped my head and said, 'Doc, don't worry about this. I'm gonna make it. I've been in worse places than this before.'"

Virgil also had a strong sense that nothing could touch him. "When I got the news that I had cancer, I was really more pissed off because it was another inconvenience in my life that I didn't really need. Growing up black in America is a challenge in itself, and this was just another impediment along the way that I just didn't need right now."

Others of us, like Charlie, remember being so ignorant of the disease that it didn't even register as an impediment. It was just no big deal. "'Oh, really!' I thought. I didn't have any information, so the diagnosis and the seriousness didn't really penetrate. I was the least-empowered human being you could ever imagine—naive to the point of absurdity and disbelief. The result was that I had absolutely no fear. I believed the doctors would fix it."

Fear wasn't in John's vocabulary either. "In many ways," he said, "I'm like Charlie. When I found out about it, I just sort of shrugged my shoulders and said, 'Well, nothing hurts, nothing bothers me.' I wasn't aware of any unusual symptoms, but that was probably because I'm a heart patient. I'm on diuretics and several other prescriptions, so I was used to urinating frequently, at different times of the day, and different ways. I'd also had one heart attack prior to my diagnosis of cancer. That was a little different, though. I knew I was having a heart attack. Prostate cancer was just two words, so I figured I would keep on going with my life as it was before."

Obviously, we all reacted differently, and that's important to remember as you read this book. How you react and how you deal with this disease and the treatments will be unique.

In retrospect, we did have one thing in common—the hidden, insidious enemy that was our lack of knowledge. We didn't have a clue what it was we *should* know, let alone be searching for. The first step for many of us was a crash course in the intimate details of

*The Prostate.*   The prostate is a small walnut-shaped gland that's located just below the bladder and surrounds the urethra. Its prime function is to manufacture part of the fluid for semen. Two microscopic bundles of nerves wrap around the outside of the prostate. These nerve bundles lead to the penis and allow you to have an erection.

One of the prime problems with the prostate is its location. As most men age, their prostate gland starts to enlarge. Because it's wrapped around the urethra, the prostate begins to compress the urethra and constrict urinary flow. Called benign (noncancerous) prostatic hyperplasia (BPH), this condition is present in about 50 percent of men in their fifties and in 80 percent of men in their eighties.

Prostate cancer takes root with a group of cells in the tissues of your prostate that do not grow, divide, or replace themselves in an orderly way. Instead, cancer cells divide rapidly and without order. These cells can form a tumor that can invade and destroy nearby tissues and organs or metastasize (spread) to other parts of the body.

Prostate cancer can grow for years with no early warning signs—or the signs are attributed to other causes, such as BPH. That's because prostate cancer often begins growing far away from the urethra. By the time the tumor starts crowding the urethra and causing problems, it's already fairly large. Unfortunately, that's one of the reasons so many men are diagnosed with an advanced stage of cancer.

Symptoms of prostate cancer include
- Weak or interrupted flow of urine.
- Frequent urination, hesitancy, or dribbling.
- Blood in the urine or ejaculate.
- Severe pain in the back, pelvis, hips, thighs.

our own anatomy. We suddenly found ourselves confronted by a double-edged sword—both our lives and our perceived sexuality were at stake.

Virgil was able to verbalize the feelings of many men, "A real man gets it up, no problem. The fear of losing that function is probably even a greater fear for some people than dying. That's why a lot of people don't want to deal with it, because if they deal with it maybe they're not going to be potent anymore. Maybe they're going to be less of a man."

*I'm going to be less of a man.* Unfortunately, that fear still keeps a good number of men away from their doctor's office, an annual exam, and, most important, a chance at early detection.

---

*DRE (digital rectal exam).* Using a gloved finger, your doctor will feel the back of the prostate gland through the rectum. If your prostate is hard or lumpy, it may be cancerous. The exam can be uncomfortable, but it shouldn't be painful and usually lasts less than a minute.

⋚⋚

*PSA (prostate-specific antigen).* PSA is an enzyme made by the prostate. It's prime function is to break down coagulated semen after ejaculation so that sperm can travel into the uterus and fertilize the egg. PSA is designed to travel out of the body during ejaculation. But any kind of infection, injury, irritation, or damage to the prostate—as well as cancer—can cause an increased level of PSA, which leaks out into the bloodstream. (The normal range of PSA is considered 0.1 to 4.0 nanograms per milliliter.) Other reasons for an elevated PSA include benign prostatic hyperplasia (BPH).

In the bloodstream, PSA occurs in different forms. For example, PSA can be "bound" or "free." Bound PSA is inactive and restrained by inhibitors from breaking down proteins. Current PSA tests detect both the bound and free molecules but don't distinguish between the two—and that would be useful. New research indicates that men with prostate cancer may have higher amounts of bound PSA than free PSA. If researchers are successful in developing more specific tests, it may be possible to distinguish PSA that's the result of prostate cancer and PSA caused by BPH.

The PSA test measures the level of PSA in your blood. The PSA test, plus information obtained from a digital rectal exam (DRE) and the use of ultrasound, can greatly increase the chance of diagnosing prostate cancer. The PSA test is not perfect, but it's the most sensitive marker of prostate cancer currently available. It's used to screen for cancer and to monitor the effectiveness of treatments.

---

"All I can say is, there I was at 10,000 feet, no parachute," remembered John. "We all know what that means. I was seeing a cardiologist because of my heart problems, and he said, 'You know,

## Research Update

Screening for prostate cancer is usually performed by a digital rectal exam and a PSA test. However, these tests and their combinations lack the specificity or accuracy needed for the selection of candidates for a further test, the prostate biopsy. Because the DRE and PSA tests do not accurately predict when a biopsy is needed, biopsies are done to confirm a diagnosis of cancer. Thus there is a high ratio between the number of biopsies performed and the number of detected cancers. To increase the specificity to predict positive prostate biopsies, the PSA test has been adjusted for prostate volume (PSA density) and age (age-specific reference ranges.)

The ratio between free and total serum PSA also improves the specificity of total serum PSA to detect prostate cancer in select patients. In a recent study, the value of the free-to-total-PSA ratio of PSAs in the intermediate range of 4 to 10ng/ml was analyzed in a screening population of 4,800 participants.

Data showed that determining the free-to-total-PSA ratio in this intermediate PSA range, or gray area, significantly improved the chances of discriminating benign from malignant prostatic diseases compared to serum PSA only. A decreased number of false-positive indications for biopsy is important, particularly in this range, since PSA values for men with benign conditions of the prostate such as prostatitis or BPH overlap considerably with those of men with malignancies. In this range, PSA-adjusted values may be helpful, since almost half of the total number of biopsies (44 percent in this study) occur in this subgroup.

The study concluded that the free-to-total-PSA ratio may be used to decrease biopsies in patients with an intermediate PSA of 4 to 10ng/ml.

Source: C.H. Bangma, J.B.W. Rietbergen, R. Kranse, B. G. Blijenberg, K. Petterson, F. H. Schroder. The free-to-total prostate-specific antigen ratio improves the specificity of prostate-specific antigen in screening for prostate cancer in the general population. *Journal of Urology* 157 (1997):2191–2196.

John, I think you ought to have a PSA test.' Well, I didn't know what a PSA was, same as a lot of you fellas. Anyway, it came back at 182. The urologist says, 'First of all, let's give you the digital on this thing.' 'Well,' I said, 'fine.' I didn't know what a digital was. I found out. He says, 'You know your prostate is smooth, pliable, no rough nodules on it. I just think you have an infection.' So he put

> *TUR or TURP (transurethral resection of the prostate).* TUR is a surgical procedure used to treat BPH. A fiber–optic instrument is placed up the urethra, allowing the surgeon to see excess prostate tissue that is blocking urinary flow. Portions of the prostate are chipped away in fragments by the instrument, through the urethra. TUR is also called the Roto-Rooter procedure.

me on antibiotics. After I finished the antibiotics, I went back for another PSA and now it was 185. So this time, he said, 'I think we'll do a biopsy.' Well, I didn't know what a biopsy was. That shows you the level of my knowledge about prostate cancer. They gave me a biopsy and found out, yes, I do have prostate cancer."

"In the summer of 1990," recalled Charlie, "my internist sent me to a urologist and he checked me out and said a TUR would take care of all my problems, and I said fine. I knew absolutely nothing about cancer. It was a negative number. It was in my vocabulary, but not much more than that. So I did the TUR, and everything was fine. I recovered and felt better. My doctor said he did a biopsy as well, and told me I was free of cancer. Cancer? I wasn't even thinking cancer. What I didn't know was that my doctor had a PSA done—and that the PSA was 29. But he never treated it, and he never mentioned it. So, a year passed. It's now the summer of '91. My wife told me about a hospital that was offering a test for men and that I ought to take it. Since I always obeyed my wife, I took it. Immediately it was Code Blue, Code Red. The bells rang. My internist shot through the phone and said, 'You've got to get right back to the urologist, right now.' I said, 'Why?' He said, 'You have a PSA of 12.' I thought, 'PSA—I wonder what that is.' So I went back to the same urologist, had a needle biopsy done—the whole bit— and discovered that I had a malignancy. And I said—'Oh.'"

"I had real problems," said Don. "I had blood in my semen. I had all kinds of scrotum problems. I had cord contractions. I could hardly walk. In fact, I thought it might be testicular cancer. When I was out shoeing horses, I noticed I was losing my power and my strength. I just felt bad. So I went to a couple of M.D.'s. They took my blood pressure, but they never gave me a physical, never gave me a digital rectal or anything. I had heard that I should go have a PSA and an ultrasound. I did have a PSA, which came back 0.0. I

The thought of having testicular cancer is certainly not funny. But a related subject precipitated an eruption of laughter when Don told us all how to "candle" testicles. For some of us it was a matter of city boy meets country boy. Here's how it went:

**Don:** I don't know if you guys know how you test your testicles or not, but I'll tell you how. You go into a dark room with a flashlight, and you candle them just like you do eggs. Have you ever candled eggs with a light? You can test your kids that way. If they're football players or whatever, you just go in a dark room and candle those testicles. If there's a spot in them, you can see it just like you would an egg.

**Virgil:** Wait a minute—not a real candle?!

**All of us:** No! They just call it candling! We want that in the book!!

was told it was about as good as it gets, which was a relief, so I decided to bypass the ultrasound for the time being. So I went about my business on through the summer and into fall. But I started having problems again and went back to my doctor. I had another blood test and a PSA, and this time it came back 2,448! They told me that within a year I'd probably have cancer in my shoulder, in my brain, and my lungs."

Whereas some of us had some warning signs, most of us felt perfectly fine. There was nothing "wrong" with us. We, too, were busy living our lives, enjoying our families, and making plans for the future. Until one day changed everything—a day that's burned into all of our brains forever.

"In July of 1993, I decided to have a routine physical exam," Bob told us, "because I planned to retire from my job as a Los Angeles police officer after 21 years. I was feeling fine. I didn't have any problems and expected no surprises from the exam. I got a big one. I had a digital rectal exam, a PSA test, and a subsequent biopsy of my prostate. My PSA was 8.5 and my stage was B1. On August 11, over the phone at work, I was told I had cancer. I was numb. I didn't know anything about prostate cancer, and the diagnosis hit three days before my wife's birthday. Needless to say, we canceled the birthday plans as well as a trip to Europe we had been planning. Suddenly, my retirement looked pretty bleak, and all my plans were disintegrating before my eyes. The following morning I drove the 35 miles to work in somewhat of a trance. I didn't have a clue what I would do next."

---

## Research Update

Current data show a decline in the incidence of prostate cancer. However, there is still a large geographic variability in incidence rates. Researchers have suggested that the variability in rates may be due to the inconsistency in screening for prostate cancer and detection of the disease.

Researchers in the Seattle–Puget Sound region evaluated this hypothesis by examining trends in the region over a span of 21 years. Analysis was restricted to white and African American men who were 35 years or older and who were diagnosed between 1974 and 1994.

The results showed the incidence of prostate cancer increased slowly from 1974, peaked in 1991, and declined in 1994. Overall, the incidence rate in the Seattle–Puget Sound region is higher than the rate in some other regions of the country, but researchers say this is likely due to more intense PSA screening of the population in this region.

The recent decline in incidence suggests that many prevalent cases of prostate cancer in our population have now been diagnosed. This pattern may also be related to changes in access to health care and health care reform in screening programs for the early detection of disease.

One of the most striking observations in the data was the 60 percent reduction in the incidence of advanced-stage prostate cancer during 1987–1997. This finding suggests that prostate cancer screening has led to a shift toward earlier-stage diagnosis, when the disease is most likely to respond to treatment, and emphasizes the importance of continued monitoring of prostate cancer mortality.

Source: L. M. Newcomer, J. L. Stanford, B. A. Blumenstein, M. K. Brawer. Temporal trends in rates of prostate cancer: Declining incidence of advanced-stage disease, 1974–1994. Journal of Urology 158 (1997): 1427–1430.

---

According to Manuel, his future looked pretty bleak, too. "For the past two years my wife and I had been remodeling a house that we bought, which was nearly in ruins. It was our pride and joy. We moved in, and the week we moved in I got the diagnosis: CANCER!! I felt cheated! Life had given me the short end of the stick! Paradoxically, I felt fine. I didn't feel sick. Fortunately, I had a wife who had been nagging me and practically twisting my arm to go and have a physical for about ten years. The only thing visibly wrong with me was that I had been having rectal bleeding, which I attributed to hemorrhoids. But I recoiled at the thought of having

*PAP (prostatic acid phosphatase).*   PAP is an enzyme that is secreted by the prostate gland. If cancer is present in the prostate, acid phosphatase can leak into the bloodstream. Like a high PSA, an elevated level of PAP can be a red flag that something may be wrong. This blood test, however, is far less sensitive than the PSA and is used far less often. The PAP is used more to determine the extent of an advanced tumor.

⋟⋞

*DNA Ploidy Analysis.*   This test reflects the genetic makeup (number of chromosomes) of the cells being examined. The test is performed on prostate tissue to determine how much DNA the cancer cells have. The results classify the specimen as being diploid, tetraploid, or aneuploid. Cancer cells that contain more DNA than normal cells tend to be faster growing and more aggressive (tetraploid or aneuploid). A cancer cell with two sets of chromosomes, or the amount found in normal cells, is slower growing and less aggressive (diploid). This test is not routinely run.

someone probe my rectum and rationalized that the bleeding wasn't serious even though I knew rectal bleeding was one of the seven signs of cancer. Actually, there were two precancerous polyps that had to be removed. When I had the complete physical, my PSA came back at 4.7. I had no idea what PSA meant. I had no idea what the danger zone was, what any of the numbers meant. My doctor said, 'Come back in three months,' which I did. By then my PSA had risen to 5.2, and it was then that I had a biopsy. Cancer was found in nearly all of the six biopsy cores. I had cancer everywhere, but I couldn't accept it. I began playing the denial game: 'There is nothing wrong with me. I feel perfectly fine. What if they labeled someone else's tissue samples by mistake—with my name? There is no history of cancer in my family. There is nothing wrong with me!'"

Among the ten of us, Virgil was the youngest to be diagnosed. "My story started less than two years ago, when I was 48. A friend of mind had been bugging me to get a PSA test. I said, 'Well, what for?' I had no symptoms. I felt great—no problems. I'm too young. And she said, 'Well, you're black, and that's one of the highest risk categories.' So I said, 'OK. I'll do it.' So I went and had a regular physical and came back with a PSA of 7. The doctor pointed out that the normal range is around 4. I asked, 'Should I be concerned?'

---

*Ultrasound.*  Ultrasound is the use of high-frequency sound waves to create an image. This procedure can be done either from outside your body, through your abdomen, or through your rectum (transrectal). The image produced can reveal cancerous tissue in your prostate.

≈≈

*Biopsy Using Transrectal Ultrasound as a Guide.*  If you have an abnormal DRE or an elevated PSA level, the next step is a transrectal ultrasound-guided biopsy. A special probe is inserted into the rectum that allows doctors to see the entire prostate and to detect cancers that can't be felt by a DRE. Doctors use transrectal ultrasound as a guide when performing a needle biopsy—inserting needles into the prostate to get samples. The biopsy device captures a "core" of tissue instead of just a few cells. In order to get a more comprehensive look, doctors take several samples or cores throughout the prostate—from the top, middle, and bottom of the gland. Pathologists then study the samples under a microscope and give the results to the physician.

---

He said, 'No, we'll monitor it again and don't worry about it.' But I did worry about it. I immediately flashed back to when my mother was diagnosed with stomach cancer 25 years ago. I remembered the feelings of helplessness as I watched her decline over the next few months and ultimately die. So at that point, after the PSA and the doctors said just wait a bit, I said the hell with that."

"I was having a routine exam for insurance purposes," Peter began. "My doctor did a DRE and found an enlarged prostate back in '86 and sent me over to a urologist who checked it and said that it was, in his judgment, benign. So I went back every six months or every year for several years. Finally, he decided to do a PSA just to get a baseline, and it came back 9.5. So he called me at the office and said something was wrong with the test and to please come down and take it again. So I took it again, and it was around 9.5 or 9.6. My doctor still thought that the prostate was benign. He told me of cases of PSA going as high as 24 due to BPH (benign prostatic hyperplasia) rather than a malignancy. I continued going to him for several sessions and my prostate continued to get larger, but he still deemed it to be benign. I said, 'Well, can't we do something else?' and he said, 'I don't know what else to do.' I said, 'How about another PSA test?' The test came back 14.5. Again, the urologist called me and said, 'Look there's something wrong.' So I went to my internist and said, 'Hey, is this really all they should be doing? Is there something else?' And he said, 'Certainly there is.' He sent me to a different urologist, who did an ultrasound, did the biopsies, and found the malignancy."

Paul began his story with a show of appreciation. "First of all, I'd like to thank my wife, Phyllis, for saving my life. She dragged me by the ear down to the doctor for an exam. I had been promising her that I'd have one after I finished up a big construction job I'd been working on. Like a lot of us here, I felt fine. I didn't have any symptoms but went in and got my checkup anyway in 1992. The doctor called back and said I had a PSA of 440, which didn't mean a thing to me at the time, but from then on, why, my life changed instantly. I received my diagnosis on a Friday and began follow-up testing on Monday. My biopsy revealed a malignancy and placed my stage at D1. I had a negative bone scan and negative MRI. My doctor decided to test my lymph nodes via an arthroscopic incision and found that they were positive."

"It all started for me in September of 1989," recalled Bud. "I was getting ready to leave for a reunion of the 102nd Division in Heerleen, Holland. It was the forty-fifth anniversary of when we freed their city in World War II. The day before I was to get on the plane, I was having trouble urinating. I had the urge to urinate but couldn't, and that had never happened to me before. I called my urologist and met him at the hospital, where I was catheterized to relieve the symptoms. It was painful, let me tell you. Needless to say, I didn't go to Europe. My doctor decided I should have a TURP, which I had performed, but my problems were just beginning. Three months later I had a prostate biopsy. I found out I had cancer on the twentieth day of December 1989. The doctors found a horribly enlarged prostate about the size of a small orange and weighing approximately 85 grams. My PSA was 76. I remember everything so well. It was Christmastime. The doctor said, 'You have to do something real soon. You've got a bad case and you may not be around a year from now. You've got to have surgery or radiation right away.' It was almost to the point where he wanted me to decide right then. And I said to him, 'My wife and I have got tickets to fly down to a home we have in Venice, Florida, and frankly, we're going down for a couple weeks to think it over. I'll call you back on the tenth of January, the day before my birthday, and I'll let you know what I'm going to do then.'"

Because you are reading this book, you may be in a situation similar to the ones in which we found ourselves: dealing with a diagnosis of prostate cancer and facing a dilemma. What does it all mean and what do I do next? Wading through a virtual alphabet soup of diagnostic terminology, you may feel intimidated by the complexity of cancer. Don't be. If you have the desire to learn, you absolutely can understand, and that understanding is your key to survival. When Manuel was told by a newly diagnosed man that he sounded like a doctor, Manuel replied, "Just wait three months, you'll be talking exactly like I am."

## Family Ties

Like breast cancer, prostate cancer tends to run in families and can be passed on from either your father or your mother. A recent study at Johns Hopkins University indicates that if you have a father or brother who has prostate cancer, your risk for developing the disease is two times greater than for the average American man. If prostate cancer runs in your family, it's also more likely to strike at a younger age when prostate cancer may be the farthest thing from your mind.

There's an additional link to breast cancer that you should be aware of: Men who have family members with defective forms of the breast cancer gene BRCA1 are also at an increased risk of developing prostate cancer.

Researchers at the National Center for Human Genome Research and Johns Hopkins have also discovered the first proof that a mutant gene can increase your risk for prostate cancer. This study is certain to initiate a race to find the defective gene responsible and develop a test that will determine who carries it. That test, however, is in the future and carries its own set of potential legal and ethical complications.

If you're African American, you have even more reason to be vigilant about annual exams. For some reason yet unknown, African American men have the highest rate of prostate cancer incidence in the world and also the highest rate of death. A recent study from the Walter Reed Army Medical Center says that PSA tests need to be modified and interpreted differently to better detect prostate cancer in African American men (see Table 1.1).

14

## Research Update

The majority of men with prostate cancer have no known risk factors for developing the disease, or for predicting whether their tumor will remain indolent, progress slowly, or become high grade and aggressive.

Researchers are trying to determine if variations in androgen receptors might help identify certain subpopulations of men with prostate cancer. For example, some men who undergo radical prostatectomies for clinically localized prostate cancer are found to have lymph node–positive disease.

The androgen hormone via the androgen receptor (AR) gene is necessary for the growth of the prostate and is presumed to play a role in the development of prostate cancer. The AR gene contains glutamine (CAG) and glycine (GGC) repeats that vary in length among individuals in the general population. Researchers screened clinically localized prostate cancers for mutations in the length of the CAG and GGC repeats.

Data suggested that a short CAG repeat length may be a risk factor for the development of clinically unsuspected lymph node–positive prostate cancer among men undergoing radical prostatectomies.

Researchers also determined that the average CAG and GGC repeats were significantly shorter in African Americans than in Caucasians. This finding could help explain the apparently higher age-specific reference ranges of serum PSA levels in African American men without prostate cancer compared to Caucasian men without prostate cancer. The shorter repeats could also help account for the higher incidence, higher mortality rate, and more aggressive nature of prostate cancer in African Americans.

Data showed that the odds of having an AR gene with a short CAG repeat were eight times higher in Caucasian men with lymph node–positive prostate cancer than in Caucasian men with lymph node–negative disease.

The study concluded that a short AR CAG may be a risk factor for the development of clinically unsuspected lymph node–positive prostate cancer among men undergoing radical prostatectomy. Further studies are needed to determine the relative risk of developing lymph node–positive disease among men in the general population with a short AR CAG repeat.

Source: J. M. Hakimi, M. P. Schoenberg, R. H. Rondinelli, S. Piantadosi, E. R. Barrack. Androgen receptor variants with short glutamine or glycine repeats may identify unique subpopulations of men with prostate cancer. *Clinical Cancer Research* 3 (1997):1599–1608.

TABLE 1.1   PSA Levels at Which Biopsies Are Performed

| Age | Caucasians (ng of PSA/ml) | African Americans (ng of PSA/ml) |
|---|---|---|
| 40–49 | above 2.5 | above 2.0 |
| 50–59 | 3.5 | 4.0 |
| 60–69 | 4.5 | 4.5 |
| 70–79 | 6.5 | 5.5 |

NOTE: Figures are based on the IMx test (Abbot); normal range 0 to 4ng of PSA per milliliter.

SOURCE: T. O. Morgan and S. J. Jacobsen. Age-specific reference ranges for serum prostate specific antigen in black men. *New England Journal of Medicine* (August 1, 1996).

Despite everything we've said, there is good news about prostate cancer. If caught early, it can be "cured"—meaning it will never recur. If you're living with advanced disease, your cancer can be held in check and the symptoms managed for many years. In fact, many more men are diagnosed with prostate cancer each year than will die from it. Once again, the key is early detection.

Don't let the thought of a potentially uncomfortable exam or situation paralyze you from taking action. The discomfort is temporary and brief, and the knowledge gained could save your life.

As Derek told us, "Prostate cancer runs in my family. My brother called me from Ft. Worth and said, 'I've got prostate cancer and I had it operated on.' I said, 'What the heck are you talking about, you've got prostate cancer?' I felt fine, but somewhere in the back of my head the thought of—well it's in the family and I'm older than my brother—so I decided to have a PSA. First of all, I had to fight to get the PSA, because the doctors said I didn't need it. It turned out to be 12. Being a retired weapons controller in the Air Force, I knew I needed to be in control, so I traveled to Ft. Worth for further testing and to visit my brother. I had another PSA test that was, again, 12. But an ultrasound showed no signs of cancer, and that's when my frustration levels really began rising. The doctor said, 'There's no problem. There's no cancer. You don't need a biopsy.' Well, either his machine wasn't working properly or he couldn't read the results. Anyway, even though the doctor said I didn't need a biopsy, I wanted one! In fact, I told the doctors four times, 'Give me a

> The American Cancer Society recommends that all men age 40 and
> over have an annual digital rectal exam. If you're aged 50 or over, it's
> recommended you have an annual PSA test in addition to a digital
> rectal exam. However, if you're African American or have a family
> history of prostate cancer, it's recommended that you begin all test-
> ing at the age of 40.

biopsy!' Finally, he 'shot' me eight times, and all the cores came
back with a Gleason score of 9. Now, the doctors say, 'You've got a
problem, and we need to operate immediately.'"

## Support Systems

"We need to operate immediately." Think back to when you heard
those words. Did you really hear what your doctor was saying beyond the words "cancer" or "we need to operate immediately?"
Sometimes the trauma of receiving a diagnosis temporarily cancels
out your ability to sort through and really understand the information. As Don now vividly remembers, "When they hit you with that,
you can't even think. Your mind just goes blank. And then the doctor says, 'Well, you better do this.' And most people say, 'Well, go to
it.'"

You will be facing some very important decisions, and that's why
getting support—from whomever and wherever you're most comfortable—is so important. That support could come from your partner, family, friends, or online at your computer. As John put it, "If
you're fortunate, your support starts right at home."

Most of us were fortunate, and are fortunate, to have a wife or
significant other for support—someone to talk to and someone to
offer hope. We also found that joining a prostate cancer support
group immediately after diagnosis was one of the best things we did
for ourselves, not just for the emotional support but for the information we got from talking to other men and hearing about their
experiences.

"The doctor only allows you but 15 or 20 minutes," Paul says,
"and so you can't possibly comprehend all the information necessary. This is really where the support group comes in." A support
group lets you gather knowledge about the disease and the different

*Grading.* Grading is a way of classifying how the cancer cells look under a microscope. How they look can reflect how aggressively they may behave. The cells that look the most like normal prostate cells have clearly defined borders with clear centers. These are considered to be well differentiated or low-grade and less aggressive. Cells that don't look like normal prostate cells are considered to be poorly differentiated or high-grade and more aggressive.

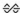

*Gleason Score.* This commonly used grading system reports the way the cancer cells look and the range of differentiation. It classifies the tumor and how aggressively the cancer cells can multiply. The Gleason grading scale goes from 2 to 10 and consists of the two most prevalent cell patterns (each pattern is graded 1 to 5) added together. For example, 3 + 4 would give you a Gleason score of 7. A score of 2 to 4 indicates low aggressiveness; a score of 5 to 6, moderate aggressiveness; and a score of 7 to 10 indicates an aggressive tumor.

If you have a high Gleason score, your cancer is more likely to be margin positive—cancer cells were found on the edges of tissue cut out during surgery. That means that cancer has probably penetrated or escaped the prostate capsule, and there is a higher chance that the cancer may have spread to the lymph nodes. Margin negative means that cancer cells were not found on the edges of tissue removed. Your cancer is probably still located within the prostate and has probably not spread to other organs.

*Staging.* Staging is a system that classifies where the cancer is located, as well as if and how far it has spread. Staging will allow you and your doctor to discuss outcomes of various treatments and, when combined with your Gleason score, to determine the most appropriate treatment. There are two similar staging systems: the Tumor Node Metastases (TNM) classification, which is preferred, and the Whitmore-Jewett system. You can easily convert from one to the other.

The Tumor Node Metastases (TNM) classification is an international staging system that combines information about the extent of the tumor (T) in the prostate gland, the involvement of the lymph nodes (N), and whether it has metastasized (M) to other organs.

The Whitmore-Jewett System also evaluates the extent of the tumor, lymph node involvement, and if the cancer has metastasized to other organs. This system uses ratings from A through D.

| TNM Classification | Whitmore-Jewett System |
|---|---|
| T = Tumor | |
| T0—reflects no evidence of primary tumor | A1 |
| T1—clinically nonapparent; tumor cannot be felt by DRE or seen by imaging | A2 |
| T1c—tumor is identified by needle biopsy because of elevated PSA only | |
| T2—Palpable tumor (tumor can be felt by DRE and is confined within the prostate gland) | |
|     T2a—tumor limited to half of one lobe or less | B1 |
|     T2b—tumor spread to half of one lobe but not to both lobes | B2 |
|     T2c—tumor spread to both lobes | B3 |
| T3—tumor penetrates wall of prostate, for example, into seminal vesicles | |
|     T3a—unilateral extracapsular spread | C1 |
|     T3b—bilateral extracapsular spread | C2 |
|     T3c—tumor spread to one or both seminal vesicles | C3 |
| T4—tumor fixed (doesn't move around easily) or grown into nearby tissues other than the seminal vesicles | |
| | |
| N = Node (the number that follows the N describes tumor spread into the lymph nodes) | |
| N0—no lymph node involvement found | D1 |
| N1—tumor found in one lymph node and is less than 2 centimeters | |
| N2—tumor found in one lymph node and is larger than 2 centimeters or more than one lymph node involved | |
| N3—tumor found in any lymph node larger than 5 centimeters | |
| M = Metastasis (the number that follows the M describes where the tumor has spread to other organs) | |
| M0—no spread outside the pelvic area (no distant metastasis) | |
| M1—tumor spread to another organ or tissue, for example, bone or a lymph node outside the pelvis (distant metastasis) | D2 |

treatment options before you make a decision about your situation. Before you make any decision, you'll need to become intimately familiar with how prostate cancer grows, or, as Virgil would say, "the nature of the beast."

Prostate cancer is made up of many different kinds of cells. Some prostate cancer cells are dependent on androgens, or male hormones, to grow; other cells, called androgen-independent cells, do not require hormones. Testosterone is the most common androgen that causes hormone-dependent prostate cancer to grow, and it is produced mainly by the testicles. Small amounts of other androgens are produced by the adrenal glands. Many of your treatment options are geared to controlling the amount of testosterone in your body or shutting down androgen production altogether.

The important thing, and you'll hear this a lot from us, is to take the time to digest your diagnosis and develop your game plan. In most cases, you do not have to make an immediate decision about treatment. Ask a lot of questions and make sure you understand the answers.

However, when you're confronted by your own mortality, the thought of leaving loved ones behind and making sure they're provided for can override all other thoughts and plans, at least in the beginning. It's a buffer zone, some would call the twilight zone, between *I'm going to die* and *I'm going to live*.

Bob remembers it this way: "I was ready to cash in and do what I needed to get my business in order for my family. I just thought that was the end of everything and all my plans and so forth were down the tubes."

With a wife and young son, Peter says he also felt an obligation to get his affairs in order. "One of the things I did when I was first diagnosed was to sell our motor home and a boat. I spent tons of time with my insurance agent. I went to my lawyer and redid wills, all in expectation that sometime in the near term, I wouldn't be here. I also owned and operated a business that I'd been president of for 15 years, and my wife worked with me in the business but she had never run the business, and here I'm thinking, 'I'm going to die.' This was our major asset and protection for her, and for our then eight-year-old son. So I resigned as president and trained my wife to run the business, and it's worked out very well for us. (I remained chairman of the board.) Other concerns I had as I was thinking of a shortened life—and I didn't know how short—was this eight-year-old youngster, and that continues to bother me; the idea of not being here when he graduates from high school or from college."

Don put it succinctly: "You wonder about your grandsons."

## Lessons in Humility

It's probably crystal clear by now that receiving a diagnosis of prostate cancer hit all of us and our families right between the eyes. But that's not the only thing that knocked us cold. How we received that diagnosis is a sore spot for many of us and sparked some heated discussions about the compassion, or lack thereof, of the medical community. And it wasn't just the actual words "you have cancer" that hit hard. What led up to that diagnosis was a real education and sparked some enlightened discussions.

"We all talk about our self-image and who we think we are," Virgil explained. "There's probably no more humiliating process than the diagnosis of prostate cancer. I mean, I never got so tired of so many guys crawling up my butt, giving me a DRE; nurses like vampires taking blood from me. I don't know if you've ever had the cystoscope. That's another thing that leaves you totally devoid of any human dignity. A fiber optic is inserted into your penis and pushed up to the prostate. I felt stripped and abused by that procedure. Afterwards, you're lying there and they dump water over you to wash everything off, and then everybody goes off to lunch. And you're there like the Gauls who've gone through Rome, and you're what's left over. You wind up getting treated as an organ, or as a disease, as opposed to a person. And it just continues to progress along the process until you finally make a decision and say this is what *I'm* going to do."

"My wife helped me with this," continued Bob. "She said we men have an attitude. We take the posture that we don't want to be examined. We feel like we're being violated when we go there. The doctor says, 'OK, bend over and spread your cheeks,' whatever, and if it's a woman doing it, it's just demeaning, or so we think. You don't want this to happen to you. It's like you said, Virgil, there were so many people going up my butt, I thought it was a freeway."

"I hear what you're saying," commented Manuel, "and what you said is OK, but you have no choice. That's part of the process of being diagnosed. You have to adjust to it. Either that or you're a dead man."

## For the Messenger

We all agreed that the "process" is a necessary evil and that any discomfort from the tests, whether physical or psychological, will pass. We also agreed that during the process, there's a need for sensitivity from the medical community, and that need often gets shelved, forgotten, or simply goes unrecognized. Maybe doctors suffer from a lack of sensitivity training or adopt a dispassionate attitude to protect themselves—to keep their emotions out of the cold war on cancer. But the fact is that many times the diagnosis is brutal. That is inexcusable and something no patient should have to endure.

Manuel remembers his doctor leaving a message on his answering machine. "The doctor said, 'I want you to call me *today*!' When he said the word 'today,' I *knew* that I had cancer. So I went back with my wife for a consultation about choosing treatment, but I sensed that my doctor was annoyed that my wife wanted to be there. You could see the annoyance. I felt that he was thinking, 'How dare you bring this woman in!' Then he would only talk directly to me, and he would talk to me like this: 'Oh yes, Mr. Vazquez, you have cancer.' He was writing in his chart as he talked. 'You have cancer and you can do three things. You can do nothing and you will die'—all the while he's reading and writing in my chart without any eye contact. 'You can have radiation and have a 70 percent chance of a cure and a 30 percent chance of being impotent or incontinent or both. Or you can have surgery and have the same situation. However, because your life expectancy is greater than ten years, if you have radiation the cancer may come back. Which one would you like?' I felt like a rug was pulled out from under my feet. Now, I have respect for the man. I think he's a good technician. He never lied to me and he told me what my options were. I knew it was up to me to make a decision, but I had a big problem with the way the message was delivered. The message was delivered like I was a dog or a cat or a machine, not a human being. It was devastating to me, absolutely devastating. This is a life-altering message and many physicians are not aware of their insensitivity when they deliver it."

Don recalls that his diagnosis was equally devastating and definitely not private: "When I was sitting in the waiting room, they said, 'Oh Mr. Zank, you've got to get another PSA. Yours is 2,448'—and it was announced over the microphone! I would have liked to have run out of the place. Anyway, I went back into the exam room and got on the table. The doctors start doing a biopsy and ultrasound, and they started pointing and saying, 'Oh man, look there, look there.' I didn't know what they were talking about. When I left the office, I knew I had cancer, but I wasn't really aware of it. I didn't know what was going on. So I went on back to work."

Most of us had legitimate gripes about our doctor's style of delivery. Paul had his horror stories as well, but as he pointed out, "It's natural to want to take a shot at the messenger that brought the bad news. By the same token," he went on to say, "we have to appreciate these doctors who've spent a lot of time and effort learning to get where they're at. We need to try to do the things to get the most information out of them—information that's going to be of benefit to us."

In other words, if you're going to fight this disease, you're going to need good working relationships with your health care providers, and those relationships need strong foundations right from the start. Remember, it's your life, so if you're uncomfortable with your doctor, or doctors, or can't talk with them, first try some of the techniques you'll read about in this book. They may help you to educate your doctors on the type of relationship you need. If this doesn't work, you might want to find another physician.

What advice would we give to health care professionals? Plenty.

Bob says, "First and foremost, remember the Golden Rule—how you would like to be treated. If the doctors did that, why, maybe they'd have a little more consideration. As a patient with a problem, I think that you should take a proactive approach with your doctor. I've 'trained' my doctor somewhat, because I gave him a good lashing: 'You will *not* talk to me this way. I am paying your salary, you are working for me. I'd like to have a more thorough approach and a more sensitive approach because this is my life and it affects me.' The bottom line? Exercise some medical compassion."

Peter agreed that medical information must be delivered with compassion but added knowledge to the equation. "The compassion, I think, comes from two things. One is training as a medical student on how to be compassionate. That needs to be incorporated somehow in training by imbuing them with a level of sensitivity. Somehow, they need to remove the defenses that they need to survive every day."

Charlie was quick to point out, "The communication of your health status in most cases comes from a urologist, initially. What they are missing in their training is communication. They need to be

# Research Update

In 1997, based on revised projections, prostate cancer will be diagnosed in an estimated 209,000 American men; 41,800 will die of the disease, making it the second leading cause of cancer death in men after lung cancer. Prostate cancer accounts for 36 percent of all male cancers in the United States and 13 percent of cancer-related deaths in men.

The incidence of prostate cancer is 66 percent higher among African American men than among white men. In fact, African American men experience the highest prostate cancer incidence rates in the world, and associated mortality rates are twice those of white men.

The study also says that no direct evidence exists to show that PSA screening decreases prostate cancer mortality rates. Indirect evidence, however, suggests that prostate cancer screening has resulted in the diagnosis of earlier-stage disease in more younger men, which could influence mortality.

Based on data from ongoing clinical trials, the American Cancer Society has updated its guidelines on prostate cancer screening. In 1997, the ACS recommended that both the PSA test and the digital rectal exam (DRE) be offered annually, beginning at age 50 to men who have a life expectancy of at least ten years. Men who are in high-risk groups, such as those with a strong familial history (e.g., two or more affected first-degree relatives) or African Americans may begin at a younger age (e.g., 45 years). More data on the precise age to start prostate cancer screening are needed for men at high risk.

The updated guidelines emphasize the need to give patients more information about the risks and benefits of intervention. For example, the ACS now recommends that physicians inform prostate cancer patients that a PSA value less than 4ng/ml does not guarantee that cancer is not present, because up to 25 percent of men with the disease can have PSA levels of less than 4.

Men whose screening results are positive are faced with the difficult decision of whether to submit to curative therapy such as a radical prostatectomy or radiation treatment and the accompanying risks. The rising incidence of prostate cancer that has resulted from more ambitious screening efforts has already led to an increase in the number of radical prostatectomies and radiation treatments performed in the United States.

Source: A. von Eschenbach, R. Ho, G. P. Murphy, M. Cunningham, N. Lins. American Cancer Society guideline for the early detection of prostate cancer: Update 1997. *CA: A Cancer Journal for Clinicians* 47 (1997):261–264.

> For the Messenger:
>
> • Treat us as you would like to be treated.
> • Deliver the diagnosis with respect and compassion.
> • Allow enough time for us to formulate and ask questions.
> • Give us as many treatment options as you can—not just your specialty.
> • Encourage us to take the time to make the necessary decisions.
> • Encourage information gathering.
> • Refer us to a support group.
> • Reinforce helpful coping styles.
> • Give us hope.

able to communicate much more information, like all treatment options and side effects, so the informed patient can make the decision. They have to get on the same level as American business. American business is spending millions of dollars to train their employees to be sensitized and to deal with an angry customer who has a problem—in other words, to discuss the problem and solve the problem."

For Virgil, the key issue is that health care providers must realize they're dealing with a person. "It's a person who has a disease, who has an afflicted organ, but in many cases, they're not dealing with the person, just with the disease. It's ultimately a person that they have to interrelate with and they have to be responsive to."

Don says he'd like to see a physician "give people all their options rather than what they sell," and Derek asks that doctors immediately send a newly diagnosed person to a support group "to get all the information."

Bud summed up the discussion, "If I were sitting in the doctor's chair, knowing what I know today, I would say to someone getting the diagnosis, 'I need to tell you, Joe or John, you've got prostate cancer. That's the bad news. The good news is that we have so many good ways to treat it today.'"

With knowledge comes empowerment, and with empowerment comes hope.

# 2

# *Decisions*

## THE LEARNING CURVE

*The more I found out about prostate cancer and the alternatives
and the treatments for it, the less fear I had of it.*
—*Bob White*

It was not a bad dream. We all woke up the morning after the diagnosis to the blunt reality of having cancer. So now what? Most of us barely knew where our prostate was. So here we were—innocent babes in the woods. Maybe we were all still in an embryonic state of shock.

One thing we knew for sure. We knew we had treatment decisions to make. But how do you make a decision with little or no knowledge upon which to base it?

Most of us got bare-bones facts from our doctors. We found out where our prostates were and were told the basic treatment options—surgery and radiation—and some of us learned about hormonal therapy as well. But when you're completely naive about a subject, a problem quickly emerges: You don't know if you're getting all the information you need. You don't know if you're getting good, biased, or bad information. And you certainly don't know if you're getting all the treatment options so you can make a truly informed decision.

"Immediately, you find that you've got any number of counselors out there—neighbors, friends, and medical professionals—who have an opinion," Virgil says, "and they want to put that opinion on you and say that this is the only true treatment that you can go with. The things you have to resist are those well-meaning intentions that play off your emotions or your need to resolve this issue.

If you don't, you could end up choosing an improper course for yourself."

Charlie says you also have to be careful about all the preconceived notions you might have had about cancer. "Prior to the diagnosis, we already had a whole lot of impressions, but they weren't close to the surface because they didn't affect us. But then someone said, 'Hey, you have this disease'—bang! All that information that you've collected about cancer comes to the surface in a very negative way, in an untruthful way that impacts people negatively—with fear. The point I'm making is that there's a lot of information out there already. But a lot of it is bad information, or it's incorrect. And that creates or contributes to the problem of how we react to the diagnosis and how we make our decisions about treatment. Many prostate cancer patients never get the correct information, and all too many never get to empowerment, which is the key to survival."

Many factors directed our paths toward a decision. Obviously, one was our doctor's recommendation. Most of us were diagnosed by a urologist, and one thing you should keep in mind as you make your decision is that urologists perform surgery. That is their specialty and, depending on the stage of your disease, that is what they will probably recommend—so buyer beware. As Charlie passionately made clear to us, "As an attorney, I am in a major attack mode on behalf of all the prostate cancer patients in the world, and we're fighting the 12,000 urologists, many of whom deny patients' choices—by simply not telling them of all their options."

In other words, give us the whole truth and nothing but the truth. That way we can make an informed decision. Isn't that what the doctor-patient relationship should be all about?

"I think my doctors had already decided I would have surgery before they even asked," John admits. "Picture this. There are five urologists against one person with no knowledge of prostate cancer and they all agree that I should have surgery. Well, thanks to my cardiologist, they were forewarned about my condition. He told them, 'Well, you can go in and check, but please keep in mind that John is a heart patient. Consequently, you've got to approach this from the standpoint of how long can he stay on the operating table, because we want to be sure he comes out alive.' Good point!"

"Fortunately, they put me in the cardiology area in the hospital. When they opened me up during surgery, they found a three-inch tumor on the backside of my prostate, and it had already escaped into

*External-Beam Radiation.* External-beam radiation is the focused delivery of radiation to the prostate gland and surrounding tissues to kill the cancer. The treatment is given five days a week, takes about six to seven weeks to complete, and is delivered on an outpatient basis. Radiation should be delayed for four to six weeks if you have had a TURP (transrethral resection of the prostate).

Advantages:
• No surgery or hospitalization needed.
• Less impotence and incontinence than from a radical prostatectomy.
• Results and potential for a cure are similar to radical prostatectomy for the first five years.

Disadvantages:
• Daily 15- to 20-minute clinic visits for treatment—five days a week for six to seven weeks (the actual treatment lasts under five minutes).
• Possibility of impotence—usually delayed 6 to 24 months.
• Possibility of urinary incontinence.
• Possibility of bladder or rectal damage, irritation, or bleeding.
• Fatigue.
• Diarrhea.
• Skin reactions.
• Possible recurrence of cancer.

Cost: Approximately $14,000 to $20,000 (1997 estimates).

Insurance coverage: Yes.

the lymph nodes. On the fifteenth of October 1991, they took out my lymph nodes along with the tumor, but they left my prostate intact. And the only reason they didn't take it out was because they didn't think I'd live through the rest of the operation. What followed was pretty much a nightmare for me and for my wife, Rosalie. On the nineteenth, my catheter got stuck—you guys know the feeling on that—so the doctors had to go in and ream me out. And let me tell you about reaming out. It looks like they've got this big wire with a hook on it, and the doctor says, 'Boy, you can really stand pain.' I said, 'The hell I can!' But enough said on that! Then on the twentieth, I had a heart attack in the hospital. On the twenty-first, they did an angiogram, and on the twenty-second, they did a sextuple bypass on me. And each time they would go to my wife and say, 'Well, we don't think he's going to make it.' And I remember thinking to myself, 'Hey God, as long as we're here, let's get this all over with at once. Just take everything,' and I think He heard me. The reason I didn't die is I really didn't think anything about dying. I figured, heck, this is another surgery, let's go in, have it done, and see what happens. I was expecting the best—and expecting to live. I think the biggest mistake I made was deciding to have radiation."

As John and all of us will tell you, there are other options and other methods besides surgery and radiation; "at least we know about them now," says John in hindsight. "The key, really, before you go in, is you start taking notes and you put one, two, three... ten questions down and you don't leave that physician's office until all ten of these questions are answered. If that physician refuses to answer, get another one. You have no obligation to that doctor; the only people you have an obligation to is yourself and your family. This is so important. You're in the driver's seat—not your doctor. He or she may be looking for that buck, or whatever it is they're going to be after. We have to discourage that and say, 'Look, I have some knowledge on this.' And each time you see a doctor, you're gaining a little more knowledge and your questions become more technical."

So our advice to you is this: Don't stop at one opinion and don't proceed with the first treatment offered. There are a multitude of options available, both mainstream and complementary, that could apply to you. You owe it to yourself to get at least a second opinion and even a third or a fourth opinion. Learn as much as you can before proceeding with any recommendation and make sure you get all your questions answered.

But how do you know what questions to ask in the first place?! We all agreed, and we've mentioned this before, that the most important thing you can do for yourself is to join a support group—before you make a decision. In your first meeting alone, you will learn more about prostate cancer than you could ever imagine. If you find yourself saying, "I can't go and talk about my problems to complete strangers," you're not alone. A lot of us felt the same way—at first.

Manuel says his first time just felt strange! "I walked in and found a bunch of 'old' people, and for the first time in my life, I confronted the fact that I was old!"

# Research Update

Patients who choose to have external-beam radiation have additional choices, including external-beam radiotherapy planned without computed tomography (CT); whole-pelvis, small-field, or conformal therapy; conformal therapy with dose escalation; and proton-beam therapy. A recent study assessed differences in disease-specific and general health-related quality-of-life changes after treatment with different external-beam irradiation techniques.

Patients were divided into three groups based on their pretreatment field size and planning technique: whole-pelvis, small-field, or conformal. All patients had clinically localized cancer of the prostate and had not received prior prostate cancer treatment.

Measures of bowel, urinary, and sexual function and of global health-related quality-of-life parameters were obtained from self-report questionnaires. Patients completed the questionnaires before starting therapy and at 3 and 12 months after therapy. (Quality-of-life parameters are from the Health Survey Short Form [SF-36] and the Profile of Mood States [POMS].)

Data showed that irritative gastrointestinal and genitourinary side effects were frequent 3 months after treatment but had substantially abated at 12 months. Sexual dysfunction increased steadily over the study period. Despite small patient numbers, researchers found trends in favor of conformal therapy across several parameters including sexual function. In the fatigue, energy, and vigor subscales, patients who received whole-pelvis treatment fared significantly worse than those in the other two groups.

The study suggests that smaller radiation fields limit treatment-related complications and may assist patients in choosing therapy and anticipating complications. Researchers stress, however, that to compare the relative long-term quality-of-life effects of the different types of radiation more precisely, confirmation in a larger study with a longer follow-up is necessary.

Source: C. J. Beard, K. J. Propert, P. P. Rieker, J. A. Clark, I. Kaplan, P. W. Kantoff, J. A. Talcott. Complications after treatment with external-beam irradiation in early-stage prostate cancer patients: A prospective multiinstitutional outcomes study. *Journal of Clinical Oncology* 15, 1 (1997):223–229.

Paul also remembers going to his first support group meeting and deciding—on first impression—that this was not for him. "My wife, Phyllis, kindly went with me, and I was crying. I couldn't manage to stop the tears, and I said, 'Boy this is just a meeting of people who don't know how to pee or something.' That was my impression of it."

Phyllis Georgeades was one of four wives who participated in the retreat. She says that Paul was indeed devastated when he was first diagnosed. "He didn't want to talk about it at all. To get him to go to that first support group meeting was really an interesting experience because the room was a long, narrow room, and there were chairs all the way around. We got there kind of early, so we walked all the way to the end and sat back in the corner because we kind of wanted to be incognito. Well, the room filled completely up, and everyone started talking about their problems—all the medical problems, physical problems, emotional problems, sex problems, the whole range of topics. It was really an open discussion, and I remember thinking, 'What more can they talk about?!' I thought Paul was going to get on top of the table and walk out the door! He didn't say one word. In fact, they asked him two or three questions and he wouldn't say one thing. Nothing. As we were leaving he said, 'I'll never come back to this place again, ever—ever!' And he didn't go back until about two or three months later. It was shortly after his sister had died of breast cancer. So I think he realized he needed emotional support, especially. Then, when he started going to a few more meetings, he found out that urologists and oncologists also came to speak, and he was gaining knowledge about his disease—and that is when he felt like he was having some control over it."

"I actually started attending very regularly," Paul continued. "And now, I feel very akin to these people because we share something that's so very deep emotionally. I belong to a trade union, and we call ourselves brothers, but I even feel closer to the people who have this disease than I did to the fellas in my trade union who I've shared a lot of experiences with. I've gotten a lot of satisfaction in the support group, and I think I've helped a lot of other guys, too, by encouraging them to get all the facts before agreeing to any treatment."

Phyllis finished the story. "In the beginning, I think he expected that he had a few months to live and that was about it. He was going to die, period! When he found out he might have to hang around a little longer and deal with it, he thought maybe he better get something to help him along."

Bob knew that he was probably going to need some help along the way, too, and found what he was looking for—by accident. "I was reading the paper and actually saw a thing that said 'Prostate Cancer Forum Support Group' and a number to call. I called the number, and I talked with one of the facilitators, Murray Corwin. The first thing Murray told me was, 'Let me tell you that a diagnosis of prostate cancer is not necessarily a death sentence.' That was the most calming thing I could have heard at that particular time because I had given myself that death sentence and that was that. What Murray told me gave me hope. I went to the meeting and they were giving out a lot of literature, and I took everything I could—a pile of everything that was there. And I started reading and reading and reading to try to find out what is this thing that's invaded my body? What is it about? What can I do about it? The more I read, the less scared I was."

And that's what kept us coming back—"that hunger for knowledge," as Bob put it. "And the encouragement. When Murray introduced me to the group as 'that fellow who believed he had a death sentence,' they all laughed, and that was the best thing they could have done for me. I went back for more of that kind of thing—all very positive stuff, and I also quickly realized that I wasn't there as part of any age group but that I'm there because we all share something in common."

Virgil agreed with Bob. "The encouragement you got overcame any disparities in age. In fact, one of the things we were able to do, because a lot of us were younger, is guide the group toward dealing with a lot more of the emotional issues. We brought in a couple of social workers who talked about biofeedback and alternative therapies. One guy came in with laugh therapy, so we were able to get into the 'soft' side of the issue as opposed to strictly dealing with the very clinical side."

Knowledge—whether it's hard or soft—is power. And once you've tasted it, you'll wonder how you managed without it. In fact, once we got a taste of it, our lives and our outlooks began a kind of metamorphosis—from naïveté to the beginning of empowerment. But becoming empowered doesn't automatically happen or fall from the sky along with your diagnosis. You have to make the effort. Don says reading a book called *Cancer Battle Plan* by Anne Frahm was a real inspiration to him. He remembers thinking, "I can do this."

Don's wife, Lynne, says that's exactly what he did. "I'm a take-charge, controlling kind of person," she told us, "and I thought I

## Support Groups

There are several major support groups with chapters across the country. In addition, there are many more unaffiliated support groups that meet in local hospitals. Call the hospitals or the offices of the major support groups to get a referral to the group nearest you.

Man to Man
American Cancer Society
1599 Clifton Rd NE
Atlanta, GA 30329
1–800-ACS–2345
http://www.cancer.org

PAACT
1143 Parmalee NW
Grand Rapids, MI 49504
616–453–1477
Fax: 616–453–1846
http://rattler.cameron.
edu/paact

US TOO International, Inc.
930 North York Rd., Suite 50
Hinsdale, IL 60521–2993
1–800–80-USTOO
Fax: 630–323–1003
http://www.ustoo.com

Prostate Forum
Fullerton, CA 92633
714–526–3793
714–633–9241
(affiliated with PAACT,
  ACS, US TOO)

The Prostate Forum is a support group sponsored by the American Cancer Society and affiliated only with organizations that provide information, such as PAACT, US TOO, and Man to Man. Like the other major groups, it provides a forum for the exchange of information and the sharing of experiences. It is one of the largest support groups on the West Coast.

Education Center for Prostate Cancer Patients (ECPCP)
P.O. Box 948
Westbury, NY 11590
516–997–1777
Fax: 516–997–9555
e-mail: JL3730@aol.com

*(continues)*

was going to have to show him how to handle this, but everything happened so fast. I mean, the day after he was diagnosed he was at a support group. He got involved with some people the very first day, and he's been involved ever since. The people at the group were

---

**Support Groups** *(continued)*

The ECPCP is a national nonprofit organization with the goal of saving or lengthening the lives of prostate cancer patients through education, counseling, advice, and research. Advisers answer general questions about prostate cancer and offer suggestions based on current research. No phone call is turned away, but there is a suggested $50 donation to become a member. That includes a bimonthly 24-page newsletter covering conventional and complementary therapies and a monthly one-page prostate "Infogram."

For information on starting your own support group, consult the following publications:

*Living with Prostate Cancer: A Guide for Establishing Support Groups.* Zeneca Pharmaceuticals, 1994. For a copy call Zeneca Pharmaceuticals Group, Professional Relations Department, 1–800–456–3660, ext. 7862.

*Man to Man: How to Begin and Promote a Prostate Cancer Support Group* (based on the experiences of the Man to Man group of Sarasota, Florida). American Cancer Society, 1993. For a copy write or call American Cancer Society Florida Division, Inc., 3709 W. Jetton Ave., Tampa, FL 33629, 1-800-ACS–2345.

*A Guide to Establishing an US TOO Support Group.* US TOO International, Inc., 1996. For a copy write or call US TOO International (see address and phone number above).

---

very, very helpful and just reached out and supported him like he'd never seen anyone do before."

That group was PAACT—Patient Advocates for Advanced Cancer Treatment—and for many of us, including Derek and Charlie, hooking up with PAACT and its founder, Lloyd Ney, was our jump start into action. "It was Lloyd Ney and the members of PAACT who really informed me of what the options were," Charlie remembers. "They empowered me with knowledge, and the information I got from them led to whole new areas of searching. I read everything—computer reports, stacks of stuff. And it changed my whole attitude. Once I got on that track, boy, did I start to move, and I let my doctors know that I was in charge. I had the information. Unfortunately, I didn't have that attitude when I was first diagnosed."

Finding a support group changed John's attitude, too. "My wife, Rosalie, and I discovered a support group that met right in our community—a part of US TOO International," John says. "Both Rosalie and I began attending the meetings, and we found out right away that you've got this learning curve. To me, this is so important—that learning curve. And the hope and encouragement you get from hearing other people's stories. We've had people in the support group who have survived 12, 15 years. My viewpoint is that you just don't know how long you've had the cancer prior to the time you're diagnosed. We always judge we've had the tumor five or ten years before we actually discover that we have prostate cancer. In my case, they took out a three-inch tumor. How long had it been there? You don't grow a three-inch tumor overnight, so I may have already had prostate cancer five years before they told me about it. So the point I'm trying to make is that a diagnosis of prostate cancer does not mean you're going to die tomorrow."

Rosalie added some wry observations about support groups and the sexes. "We have US TOO meetings once a month, and I've noticed at the meetings that it generally takes—for men that tend to be shy—about three meetings before they really open up. By the time the man comes three times, he's able to cry, he's able to curse, he's able to hug and to kiss the men who are there. And the men are able to put their arms around him and hug him and let him know that it's OK, that it's not weak or effeminate or anything like that. It's going to be a huge educational project to get men to realize that it's healthy to cry and it's OK to share private, intimate details. And it's OK to call body parts by their proper names. When some of the women started to hear them talk about their penis, their gonads, their testicles, or all the rest of this—I thought some were going to die. You have to use the right terms and get people out of this puritanical attitude about 'you just don't discuss your private parts,' because with this disease, you have to."

Lynne agreed with Rosalie, but she also remembered a little initial discomfort. "I'm an RN, and I was even a little surprised at the frank way everyone talked—and I was shocked that I was shocked!"

Phyllis remembers thinking, "My god, what more can they talk about? But it was very informative, so I just tried to be real cool about it"—at which time Manuel chimed in, "Did they have live sex on stage?" Well, not quite.

The point is to find a good support group and join it, and there are many different kinds. As Peter says, "Support groups do not fit one standard mold." Some groups focus on psychosocial support, some on education, though most offer a balance between the two areas. No matter where you get your support and your knowledge, the main thing is getting that knowledge—good, solid information you can use to help you make your own personal decisions. "I not only go to support groups regularly," Bud says, "I was one of the early participants in the first Man to Man group in Sarasota. Then we started one in Venice, Florida, and then in Saginaw, Michigan." So if there isn't one in your area—start one!

If you own a computer or have access to one, log onto the Internet. You'll find an incredible amount of state-of-the-art information on cancer in general and on prostate cancer specifically, and you'll link into a cyber support system as well. As Virgil says, "It's the largest support group you're ever going to find." But if this is your main source of knowledge or support, don't rule out the conventional groups. Most of us are computer literate or are learning fast but still find that face-to-face encounter with real people and real emotion invaluable. Paul put it like this: "The conventional support groups, as far as I'm concerned, are the main ones because I'm looking you right in the eye."

Peter wishes he'd had the option. "I was diagnosed back in 1990," Peter remembers, "and at that time, there weren't any support groups in my area and all the informational material to go through, so I didn't have that option available, or at least I didn't know where to get the data. When I was diagnosed, I was the type of person who did what the doctor said—in the way you took the car to the garage for repair. They called me when it was ready, and I picked it up. Unfortunately, I did that through the initial diagnosis and treatment with the cancer. I'm not that person now because of what I've learned, but as far as the initial reaction, it was one of getting the diagnosis and getting the recommendation to have a radical prostatectomy. I have to say that my doctor did go through the options. He didn't just take his specialty and push it. He may have slanted it that way, but he didn't push it hard. And I followed his recommendation. I've become much more independent, critical, and more self-determining as I've acquired more knowledge about the disease and about the lack of knowledge of the doctors. And I'm now very active with the Man to Man support groups. What I've

*Radical Prostatectomy.*   A radical prostatectomy is a major surgical procedure that includes the removal of the prostate gland, seminal vesicles, any visible cancer, and a sampling of nearby lymph nodes. There are two different surgical approaches to prostate removal: retropubic (the incision is made below the navel to the pubic bone) and perineal (the incision is made between the scrotum and the rectum). During the operation, surgeons try to protect the surrounding tissues and nerves so that the patient can return to normal urinary and sexual function as soon as possible. The nerve-sparing technique to preserve sexual function is generally referred to as the "Walsh procedure" after the surgeon at Johns Hopkins who devised it.

Advantages:
• May "cure" prostate cancer in early stages (T1 and T2, A and B) when the cancer is confined to the prostate. (The patient is considered cured if he is cancer free ten years after surgery.)

Disadvantages:
• Major surgery that requires anesthesia with associated risks (including death), hospitalization for two to five days, and recovery time averaging from two to six weeks or longer depending on your individual case.
• Can cause heavy bleeding during and after surgery, usually caused by an injured blood vessel.
• Can cause blood clots.
• Possibility of infection after surgery.
• Possibility of urinary incontinence (unable to control urine), temporary or permanent.
• Possibility of impotence (unable to attain erection), temporary or permanent.
• Possible recurrence of cancer or inability to remove all the cancer; may require more treatment.

Cost: $18,000 to $23,000+ (1997 estimates).

Insurance coverage: Yes.

learned is that there's a lot that isn't known about this disease by anybody. In fact, the better the doctor, the more likely he or she is to say, 'Well, we really don't know what causes this' or 'We really don't know what the effect of this particular protocol will be.' But

## Research Update

Radical prostatectomy and external-beam radiotherapy are the two most common modalities used in the treatment of localized prostate cancer, and the comparison between the two has generated significant controversy. Researchers evaluated the outcomes after radical prostatectomy (RP) and radiation (RT) for treatment of localized prostate cancer at a single institution.

Five hundred fifty-one patients with clinical-stage T1 or T2 cancer were included in the analysis. Two hundred ninety-eight patients underwent surgery and 253 were treated with radiation. The RT patients were treated with conventional radiotherapy with standard radiation fields and doses. None of the cases analyzed received neoadjuvant or adjuvant treatment. The median pretreatment PSA level for RP patients was 8.1 versus 12.1 for the RT patients.

Two risk groups for relapse were defined using PSA and Gleason scores: low-risk (PSA < or equal to 10 and Gleason score < or equal to 6) and high-risk (PSA > 10 or Gleason score > or equal to 7). The five-year biochemical relapse survival rates (bRFS) for the low- and high-risk groups were 81 percent and 34 percent, respectively. The rate of surgical margin involvement in RP patients was 39 percent in the low-risk group versus 59 percent in the high-risk group.

By using biochemical failure as an endpoint, researchers documented more failures after RP or RT than previously suspected. (All clinical relapses were associated with rising PSA levels.)

*(continues)*

at the time, I thought that a radical prostatectomy was the way I should proceed."

In many ways, Paul's experience paralleled Peter's. "I always trusted my doctors," Paul says with a smile. "If I had a problem with my teeth, I'd go to the dentist, sit in the chair, describe my problems, and he would take care of it. I no longer had the problem—it was the dentist's problem. If I broke my leg, I went to the doctor and it became his problem, and I just did whatever he told me. I thought this was the way it went. So I stumbled along for a while and found out that it isn't the case, and if you want to survive, you better learn. But, when I was first diagnosed, that wasn't the case. My cancer was advanced when it was diagnosed. My PSA was 440 and I had cancer in the lymph nodes. I was doomed, so to speak, or at least that's how I

---

**Research Update** *(continued)*

Cases treated with RT and RP demonstrated equivalent outcomes when stratified by risk groups. For low-risk cases, the control rate exceeded 80 percent at five years with either treatment. The fact that there was no difference in bRFS rates between RT cases and negative-margin RP cases indicates that standard radiation doses are adequate to control low-risk cases. Results obtained with ultrasound-guided radioactive seed implantation are also very encouraging.

However, there were significant differences in outcomes in some patient subsets. Positive surgical margins are a predictor for poor outcome even in low-risk cases.

High-risk patients treated with radiation appeared to have higher recurrence rates after five years. Researchers concluded that failure rates were unacceptably high in high-risk patients treated with radiotherapy using standard doses and techniques. Standard radiotherapy alone should be recommended with caution in this group of patients. Good results are achieved with surgery if negative resection margins can be achieved.

For high-risk patients, several new treatment approaches are currently being investigated with either high-dose conformal radiotherapy, with or without androgen blockade, or neoadjuvant androgen blockade and radical prostatectomy.

Source: P. Kupelian, J. Katcher, H. Levin, C. Zippe, J. Suh, R. Macklis, E. Klein. External-beam radiotherapy versus radical prostatectomy for clinical stage T1–2 prostate cancer: Therapeutic implications of stratification by pretreatment PSA levels and biopsy Gleason scores. *Cancer Journal* 3, 2 (1997):78–87.

---

felt at the time. My doctor advised me to have an orchiectomy, which would slow down the cancer, so that's what I ended up doing. I was given a choice. I was informed about radical prostatectomies and was told that would be an option if my lymph nodes were negative. To tell you the truth, I didn't really know the difference and I didn't know what all the options were. Unfortunately, I didn't attend my first support group meeting until after the surgery. That's when I really started to learn."

Bud was also diagnosed with advanced cancer. In fact, he was told by his doctors that he'd be lucky to live a year and that he needed to

---

### Treating Advanced Cancer

If your cancer has spread outside the prostate, you will encounter many different opinions about how your cancer should be treated. However, most doctors will agree on one thing: The goal of treatment for advanced prostate cancer is to control the growth of the tumor and to relieve any symptoms the tumor may be causing. You and your doctor will determine your treatment choices based on your age, symptoms, general health, and whether the prostate cancer has spread beyond the pelvis.

---

have surgery or radiation immediately. He immediately decided to think it over with his wife, instead, while vacationing in Florida. "I almost came to my treatment decision by fate," he remembers. "My mother used to say, 'Don't ask for anything you want unless you're sure you want it because you're liable to get it.' And she'd add to that, 'Don't ask for something you don't want unless it's God's will.' That leaves a lot of leeway, and I think some of my Catholic upbringing is coming into this. Anyway, I went down to Florida and one of my good tennis buddies told me about two doctors—a Dr. Whitmore and a Dr. Barzell, formerly chief urologists with Sloan-Kettering and Harvard University. And my buddy said, 'These are great doctors. Why don't you go see them?' What do you call that, fate? I believe we are directed if we let our minds go. It may be a superior power or somebody helps us. So I made an appointment to go see these doctors and they said, 'We've got a new medication out, and what we understand is that from prior experience in Canada and other places, it stops the growth of cancer and it shrinks the prostate.' At that time, I had another PSA, which was up to 79 from 76, and my cancer was now staged at D1, not B2 as originally diagnosed. These doctors recommended that I go on Eulexin, a drug just recently approved by the FDA for use in the United States, and Lupron®, which had been used for several years in Canada. I felt maybe I was being a guinea pig, but I thought, 'This is for me because I need time to think things over.' I started on both drugs in January of 1990. The idea at the time was to try to shrink my en-

## Hormonal Therapy Overview

A variety of hormones are available to treat prostate cancer. They may be used alone, which is called monotherapy, or in combination, called combined hormonal therapy (CHT).

The goal of hormonal therapy is to control the level of androgens in your body—which in turn will help control, but not cure, your cancer. There are two basic ways to do this: with drugs or with surgery (bilateral orchiectomy).

To explain how hormonal therapy works, let's start with the brain. A gland called the hypothalamus makes a substance called luteinizing hormone-releasing hormone, or LHRH. LHRH acts as a chemical signal. It tells the pituitary gland to transmit another signal, called luteinizing hormone, or LH. LH tells the testicles to make testosterone.

There are different types of drug therapy. Each type targets a different area in the hormone chain of command. LHRH agonists (synthetic look-alikes of a drug or body chemical) such as Lupron® or Zolodex™ tell the pituitary to shut down LH production, thus shutting down testosterone production. The second way drug therapy works is to block or reduce the effects of other androgens at the tumor site. This is called antiandrogen therapy.

Hormonal therapy can be very effective in controlling the growth of prostate cancer. Your doctor will monitor its effectiveness by watching your symptoms and by testing your PSA levels. PSA should drop to very low levels if the hormonal therapy is working.

Although hormonal therapy is used mainly for advanced prostate cancer, drugs may also be used to shrink the tumor in early stages of cancer and may be used prior to radical prostatectomy or radiation. Because cancer cells can become hormone-resistant (androgen independent), hormonal therapy usually stops working after a period of time.

larged prostate and then consider either surgery or radiation. It was a gamble. I knew that this therapy wasn't being used regularly in the United States, but I thought it was worth a try."

What makes us try certain therapies and reject others? What factors are in play in life-and-death decisions? For some, such decisions result from a pragmatic progression of events. You look at the obvious factors in your life and then make the best decision you can with the information you have.

*LHRH agonists (luteinizing hormone-releasing hormones).* LHRH agonists are synthetic forms of a natural hormone in the body that stimulates testosterone production. Therapy using LHRH agonists tricks the pituitary into stopping production of the hormone LH. That, in turn, shuts down testosterone production in the testicles. The androgen-dependent cancer cells fail to get the hormones they need to grow.

Your doctor will give you an injection—either once a month or once every three months. Leuprolide (Lupron®) and goserelin (Zoladex™) are two hormones in this category.

LHRH agonists don't always work right away. When you begin taking this therapy, your testosterone levels can actually increase for about a week. This is called "flare," and it occurs because your body is initially confused by the type of signal the LHRH agonists are sending. Your doctor can prescribe another drug (usually flutamide [Eulexin®] or bicalutamide [Casodex®]) for the first couple of weeks to counteract the problem.

Advantages:
- Involves an injection every month or every three months with leuprolide (Lupron®) or injecting a pellet under the skin with goserelin (Zoladex™).
- Avoids surgical procedure for bilateral orchiectomy.
- Is as effective as bilateral orchiectomy as long as you take the drug.
- Effects can be reversed.

Disadvantages:
- Repeated office visits required; either once a month or once every three months depending on your medication.
- Can cause a brief increase in cancer symptoms (flare) before testosterone levels begin to fall. This flare can be minimized by taking antiandrogen pills (usually flutamide) two weeks before starting LHRH agonist therapy.
- Can cause hot flashes, breast tenderness and enlargement (gynecomastia).
- Can cause decreased interest in sex (loss of libido) and impotence.
- Psychological side effects from loss of sexual function or sense of "manliness" are possible.

Cost: Leuprolide (Lupron®), $500/month; goserelin (Zoladex™), $400/month (1997 estimates).

Insurance coverage: Yes.

*Antiandrogen therapy.* In addition to testosterone produced by the testicles, a small amount of androgens, or male hormones, are also made in the adrenal glands. Antiandrogen therapy blocks androgen receptor sites on hormone-dependent cancer cells, so the androgens cannot activate the receptors and feed the cancer. This therapy may be used alone, in combination with LHRH therapy, or after a bilateral orchiectomy.

Common drugs used in antiandrogen therapy are flutamide (Eulexin®), which requires two pills taken every eight hours; bicalutamide (Casodex®), which is a tablet taken once a day; and nilutamide (Nilandron®), which is three to six tablets taken daily. (Flutamide, bicaluatamide, and nilutamide are not FDA approved as monotherapies in the United States. They are only FDA approved if used in combination with hormonal therapy or after a bilateral orchiectomy).

Advantages:
- If used alone, may preserve potency but is inferior to LHRH therapy or bilateral orchiectomy.
- When combined with LHRH therapy, may be superior to LHRH alone or bilateral orchiectomy alone in some patients.
- Combined therapy may be of benefit before prostate surgery or before or during radiation therapy to shrink the tumor.

Disadvantages:
- Can cause diarrhea, which can usually be controlled by adjusting the dosage.
- Can cause hot flashes and breast tenderness and enlargement (gynecomastia).
- Can cause nausea and vomiting, liver damage; liver functions should be monitored regularly via blood tests.
- When used alone, less effective than combined with LHRH therapy or bilateral orchiectomy.

Cost: Flutamide (Eulexin®) and bicalutamide (Casodex®), $300/month; nilutamide (Nilandron®), $230/month. Costs vary with individual pharmacies (1997 estimates).

Insurance coverage: Yes, if you have prescription plan.

*Combination hormonal therapy (CHT).* CHT (also called total androgen blockade therapy) is the combined use of LHRH agonist therapy or a bilateral orchiectomy and antiandrogen therapy, which blocks testosterone production by the testicles and the effects of additional androgens produced by the adrenal glands. On an experimental basis, CHT is also used in combination with either radical prostatectomy or radiation to treat early-stage prostate cancer.

Some cancer specialists say that the benefit of adding antiandrogen therapy to LHRH therapy is modest. More than 22 papers have attempted to show a benefit, and there is an average 3.5 percent improvement in survival after five years. A recent large study (SWOG [Southwest Oncology Group] trial) concluded that adding the antiandrogen flutamide after an orchiectomy does not have a clinical benefit.

Note: Some support groups, including PAACT, advocate that CHT should always be used as a first line of defense to shrink the tumor, reduce your PSA levels, and give you time to plan your next level of treatment. Talk it over with your doctor.

Advantages:
• May be associated with better survival rates than LHRH or antiandrogen therapy alone.
• Therapy lowers PSA levels in 99 percent of patients.

Disadvantages:
• More expensive than either bilateral orchiectomy or LHRH therapy alone.
• Side effects include hot flashes, fatigue, breast tenderness and enlargement (gynecomastia)—though much less than with antiandrogen therapy alone. (The antiandrogen flutamide has been associated with serious liver damage. Discuss the other side effects of antiandrogens with your doctor.)
• Decreased interest in sex; impotence likely.
• Long-term use may cause decreased muscle mass and bone loss, increased amount of fat tissue.
• Some studies show that there is no clear benefit by adding antiandrogen therapy.

Cost: $700 to $800/month (1997 estimates).

Insurance coverage: Check your insurance for antiandrogen coverage.

Mary Vazquez, Manuel's wife, added, "We talked it out a lot. We measured the pros and cons and he did a lot of the research on the Internet. He would ask me what I thought, but I think he almost knew from the very beginning that he was going to go ahead and have the RP. He is the type of personality that, when he believes in something or sets his mind to something, that's usually the way it goes. But he was terribly concerned about the possibility of incontinence and impotence—and extremely concerned about the impotence. It was very important to him."

"The hardest part," Manuel remembers, "was to pick up the phone and schedule my surgery. I literally had to force myself to do that."

Besides taking into account the things that Manuel did, such as age, stage of disease, and side effects, there are many other factors that can affect how you approach this disease. We quickly found out in the course of this retreat that our backgrounds, our ethnicities, and our occupations often dictated our course of action—or at least influenced it heavily. Very likely it will be the same for you.

"Occupation did it for me," Derek told us. "I'm retired Air Force. I spent 22 years as a fighter weapons controller, and I was definitely empowered for what I did. I knew I had to have control. I knew I had to know more about what was there before I started the fight. That was my job. I was always looking for perfection—get the radar set better; check to make sure it's at its peak. I also designed a lot of systems in my job—what's the best way to shoot? How long is it going to take? What will best get me from here to there? You're always thinking about alternatives. If someone told me I couldn't do that, I said, 'The hell I can't' and would design a system that worked. So my mind was constantly working. There's a way to do this—a way to knock your enemy down, and that's how I approached my cancer. The first step was to visit my brother, Bill, in Ft. Worth, who also had prostate cancer. Bill had undergone a radical prostatectomy, and his doctors told me that I should also have surgery. But I started reading a bit, checking things out, and I discovered that I didn't like what the doctors had done to my brother. They had cut him open, found that the cancer had spread to the lymph nodes, and they took his prostate out anyway! And my brother was suffering a lot. He was incontinent and impotent, and he was just going nuts. So surgery scared the hell out of me, and I told the doctors that they were not going to cut me open. With that, I managed to piss off the doctors in Ft. Worth and in Albuquerque, where I was first diagnosed. So basically, nobody's talking to me. I just felt like everyone was trying to push me around and strip me of my power—and I wasn't getting enough information. So I traveled to the large cancer center in Houston for a third opinion. They did another ultrasound, and during the procedure, I heard the urologist telling the radiologist how bad it looked. The opinion was the same: 'We have to operate.' So I started asking the doctor questions. 'Do you use the nerve-sparing technique?' (I had talked to Dr. Walsh's office at Johns Hopkins.) 'What kind of procedure do you use? What kind of equipment do you use? Has it all been checked out? Do you know what you're doing?' All this time the doctor's sitting there with his feet up on the desk (while I'm in a damned open-backed gown with my buns on a cold metal table), saying, 'No, we don't use nerve-sparing. We just get the job done and whatever's wrong, we'll fix it later.' Then I asked him how much time he thought that I had left, and he said that if I didn't do anything right away, I'd be dead in two years. So I responded with 'Well, of those two years, let's take two minutes to discuss other options that might be available to me. He waved that off and indicated that there was no need for that and that I should just go down the hall and give my first pint of blood for the operation. At that point I said, 'Gimme my pants, I'm outta here.' To make a long story short, I was frustrated as hell. So I literally embarked on a cross-country search for information and satisfaction. I talked to and visited more than ten universities, hospitals, and clinics from New Mexico to Michigan and New England to Florida about surgery, radiation, cryotherapy, and hormonal therapy. I had heard horror stories about guys being 'burned' with radiation, and I wasn't sure the equipment was any good, so I said 'no way' to that! I was leaning towards cryo, but I was still having a hard time because I couldn't get really comfortable with anything. But I didn't have it all solved because I still wanted combined hormonal therapy before I did anything else. The problem here was I couldn't get a doctor to prescribe it for me. In the meantime, I was getting very tired and desperate because my PSA was rising, so I finally told myself enough was enough. I walked into the radiation clinic of a large, prominent hospital that I had visited previously and explained to them (actually I lied) that I was interested in radiation but that I wanted Lupron and flutamide to stop my

*Cryotherapy.* Cryotherapy is the controlled freezing of the prostate gland to kill cancer cells. Using transrectal ultrasound as a guide, doctors circulate extremely cold liquid nitrogen through about five probes placed in the prostate gland through the perineum. An "iceball" forms and, then, as the prostate gland is allowed to thaw, the cancer cells within the gland rupture and die. A catheter inserted into the penis protects the urethra with heat. The procedure is performed with the patient under anesthesia.

Advantages:
• Minimally invasive surgery; the procedure takes about 1 hour or longer and the hospital stay is 1 to 2 days.
• Causes less incontinence.
• Treatment can be repeated.
• May be performed if cancer recurs after radical prostatectomy or radiation. Check with your doctor, however, because this is not always an option.
• Surgery or radiation may be used if cancer recurs after cryotherapy.

Disadvantages:
• Risks associated with anesthesia.
• Short-term bladder irritation.
• Temporary penile or scrotal swelling.
• Can cause impotence but rarely causes incontinence.
• No five- and ten-year survival statistics.

Cost: $10,000 (1997 estimates).

Insurance coverage: In 1996, the American Urological Association recognized cryotherapy as no longer investigational or experimental as a result of a PAACT initiative. However, private insurance companies and Medicare are still denying claims. Check with your insurance company.

Note: Administrative law judges of Medicare are approving cryotherapy. LAC-PAACT (the legal arm of PAACT) has worked with one of its member legal firms to sue Medicare in federal court on a ruling denying payment for cryotherapy. That case is active and pending.

## Research Update

Cryosurgical ablation of the prostate, also known as cryotherapy, is enjoying renewed interest, but it is not without side effects. The reported rates of incontinence and urinary retention, however, vary widely depending on whether cryotherapy is performed as a primary procedure or a salvage procedure after the primary treatment has failed. In a long-term study, researchers followed 143 patients who underwent cryotherapy after radiation therapy failed.

Data showed that incontinence and urinary retention rates are much greater in patients undergoing cryotherapy after failure of radiation therapy. Prior radiation therapy probably causes microvascular changes that exaggerate prostate tissue damage. Similarly, a damaged vascular supply to the sphincter may undermine the healing process.

The study also says that an effective urethral warmer is crucial in minimizing postoperative urinary retention and long-term incontinence. If an effective urethral warmer is used, spontaneous resolution of the problem occurs in half of the patients within one year of having the procedure performed.

The study recommends waiting at least 12 months after cryotherapy before treating incontinence because tissues usually begin to improve after 12 to 15 months. Treatments using collagen injections, for example, are much easier and more successful the longer one waits after surgery.

Source: R. D. Cespedes, L. L. Pisters, A. C. von Eschenbach, E. J. McGuire. Long-term follow-up of incontinence and obstruction after salvage cryosurgical ablation of the prostate: Results in 143 patients. *Journal of Urology* 157 (1997):237–240.

PSA from rising and to give myself some time to decide what I wanted to do. Thedoctor said that he would not recommend doing it that way, but if that was what I wanted to do, he'd write the prescriptions. I grinned as I walked out the door with a six-month prescription and said to myself, 'I'm on my way.' It had taken me almost a year to get what I wanted. Six months after I started on the CHT, I decided on cryotherapy. It seemed the least complicated, and I figured what damage can you do with a goddamn iceball? The bottom line is—right or wrong—you gotta get control!"

For Virgil, getting control simply meant getting the cancer out of his body. "My attitude was search and destroy, that's it," he says.

*3-D Conformal Radiation Therapy.*  3D conformal radiation therapy is a special external-beam radiation that more accurately focuses the radiation on the prostate cancer, thus reducing damage to nearby normal tissue. 3-D conformal therapy is custom-designed for each patient. It uses a series of CT images of the prostate, bladder, rectum, and so on to build a three-dimensional image of the area. In addition, each patient has a special body cast made to minimize movements and to duplicate the exact position during each treatment. Computers calculate the dose of radiation—segment by segment—and shape the radiation beam so that it focuses precisely on the tumor.

3-D conformal therapy allows doctors to deliver higher doses of radiation to the cancer, which have been shown to lower relapse rates. In contrast, conventional radiation is not quite as precise and may not supply enough radiation to kill the entire tumor. Also, if you increase the dosage in conventional radiation, it can result in more serious side effects.

Proton-beam radiation therapy is a less widely available type of external-beam radiation therapy that also focuses radiation more accurately on the cancer and at higher doses—minimizing damage to normal tissue.

Advantages:
- Higher doses or more precisely delivered radiation can be administered.
- There are potentially fewer and milder side effects than with traditionally delivered or planned external-beam radiation.

Disadvantages:
- Proton-beam radiation is performed at only two centers in the United States: Loma Linda University Medical Center in Loma Linda, California and Massachusetts General Hospital in Boston, Massachusetts.
- 3-D conformal therapy is more available than proton-beam therapy but is still restricted to select research-based institutions.
- No five- and ten-year survival statistics available.

Cost: Proton-beam radiation: $35,000 (1997 estimates); 3-D conformal radiation: check with your institution.

Insurance coverage: Check with your insurance carrier.

Note: Neutron-beam radiation therapy is available only at Wayne State University in Detroit, Michigan, the University of Washington in Seattle, Washington, and the Fermi Lab in Aurora, Illinois (1997). It is effective only in some types of tumors, and its use in prostate cancer is controversial. It is associated with more side effects than either 3-D conformal or proton-beam therapy.

"Now that I know who the enemy is, we're gonna get the sucker. That attitude is somewhere in my personality, I guess, but it was probably heightened in the military, in the financial industry, and in the garment industry, where I've spent a lot of time. The garment or textile industry is an industry that eats its young. You have to be able to be very hard, very cold, very calloused. You project a very macho image, and those are just the women! The attitude there is that nothing's going to touch me. I'm not going to deal with it—much like the financial industry. I work with a lot of guys on Wall Street, too, which is, again, a very macho-oriented environment that doesn't allow for the potential of weakness of any kind, much less illness. I'm also a knowledge freak. I wanted to find out as much as possible about the disease. What was it? How does it work? What are the options?

"I called Lloyd Ney and got some information from PAACT, called the American Cancer Society, got on the Internet, and started researching it extensively. I went through a whole list of options, both traditional and alternative—all in terms of how am I going to deal with this? Finally, I did a whole spreadsheet analysis, and it came down to the fact that the only thing that made sense in my condition, since everything was totally confined to the prostate, was do the surgery and get it over with. I thought that it was the best move in terms of getting rid of the cancer now. I don't look at it as necessarily curing cancer, because I don't think we know enough about it to say we've beaten it. But in terms of various therapies, I wanted it out of me. I didn't want the radiation and be left thinking that maybe they got all the cancer—maybe. I didn't want to have it still in there playing around. It may pop up again sometime or other, but at least this little bastard is not going to be there. The doctors said the radical prostatectomy is the gold standard. It's a 15-year stint for a 'cure.' Fifteen years—cancer free, I hope. [Some doctors define cure as being ten years cancer free; the National Cancer Institute percentages are based on five-year survival.] In 15 years, I'll be 65, ready to retire and get Social Security. Maybe I'll have another surprise waiting. I don't know. But I don't care either because I'll fight the battle as I have to fight it. I'm not going to worry in advance. Ultimately, I think what we have to do is clearly a matter of empowerment. Because I had taken control of my life early on, I had a very clear understanding of who I was and who I wanted to be and how I wanted to live my life. It just made my diagnosis of cancer that much easier to deal with."

---

*Saw Palmetto.*   Saw palmetto is a palm tree native to the Atlantic coast of North America. Extract from the berries (the fat and sterol portion of the berry) is thought to help reduce the size of an enlarged prostate. It is used mostly to treat benign prostatic hyperplasia (BPH).

*Watchful Waiting.*   Watchful waiting is also referred to as observation, surveillance, or deferred therapy. Basically, no treatment is given, but your doctor will continue to carefully monitor you and your tumor with frequent prostate exams and PSA tests. Treatment can be started at any time. If you have a small, low-grade cancer or if you are older or have other health problems, this may be an option for you.

Advantages:
• No treatments with their associated inconveniences or risks.

Disadvantages:
• May miss opportunity for remission possible with other treatments.
• Psychological aspect of observation is sometimes the hardest—knowing that you have cancer but are doing nothing "active" about it.

Cost: Varies.

Insurance coverage: Depending on your carrier, doctor visits and PSA tests may be covered.

---

As far as macho professions go, Bob lived one for years. It, too, programmed him to want and keep complete control. "There can be no more macho occupation than being a police officer," he says. "You are invulnerable—nothing can touch you. You can rise above any situation. You're equipped and trained to be able to handle it. You will eradicate it. It's really somewhat of a military approach because we get the same kind of conditioning. You don't talk about your illness. You go to the gym and work your way through it. You got aches and pains—you don't wimp, you don't cry, because you are an officer of the law, and you're bigger than God. You actually believe this stuff. So my occupation had a lot to do with my early denial. I'm going to beat this thing. I don't want to believe I've even got it. Now I'm at a place where I recognize the fact that I am vulnerable, and why *not* me?

Once you accept that fact, then you're open and you become a sponge, and you start soaking up all the information to try and get yourself empowered. You recognize the fact that you're a human being and these things can happen to you, too. Once you do that, I think you're on the road to actually healing yourself and taking real control.

"I consulted several urologists," Bob continued. "My first urologist wanted to give me the gold standard, a radical prostatectomy, which I refused to do. I didn't think that was the way to go for me—never did. My next urologist, who also happened to be the chief urologist at my hospital, told me, 'If I had prostate cancer, if it were me, I wouldn't do anything.' Well, that kind of scared me—doing nothing at all, so I didn't think I was ready for that either. So I kept checking around and reading about each and every procedure. I heard about 'watchful waiting,' and I thought, 'Well, that's not really doing nothing,' but it turns out that that's what I ended up doing. In fact, I did watchful waiting for the next year and a half while I continued to educate myself about all the different procedures. In the meantime, I also took saw palmetto, which began slowly lowering my PSA. After careful consideration, my first inclination was to go for the seed implants because it seemed less invasive. I consulted with Dr. Takeda at St. Joseph's Hospital in Santa Monica, who was one of the leading physicians using this procedure. He showed me figures that it had been very effective over a number of years—nothing over five or six years, though. I also went down to San Diego and talked to a doctor who does cryotherapy, got some material, and read up on that.

"In the meantime, my family was starting to get wind of the fact that I had prostate cancer. Remember, I was still in a semistate of denial. Anyway, a couple of my daughters who lived up north and my son in New York converged on me at home—my wife had told them. They were ready for—I don't know what. They had these long faces, and my young daughter was crying. They were all saying, 'What are you going to do?' and I said, 'Well, I'll tell you. I've been checking and I found out there's a lot of other alternatives that I've been looking into.' I started showing them all the literature I had and reading all the information to them. I told them I had looked at external radiation. I had also looked at the proton-beam radiation, but it was awfully expensive and I didn't think my insurance would cover it anyway. To make a long story short, after going all the way around the mulberry bush on this thing and looking at all of the options, I came back to seed implants because it was, again, the least invasive, and be-

## Research Update

Treatment for clinically localized prostate cancer remains controversial. There are several options including radiation therapy, surgery, and observation with hormonal treatment when the disease progresses. Part of the controversy arises from studies of prostate cancer that suggest patients with localized disease rarely die as a direct consequence of their malignancy regardless of treatment.

In a recent study, researchers tried to evaluate the impact of radiotherapy and to determine 15-year survival and recurrence rates after internal and external-beam radiation for localized prostate cancer.

One hundred thirty-six patients with clinically localized disease were treated from 1966 to 1974 with interstitial gold seed (brachytherapy) and external-beam radiation and were evaluated. No patients received hormonal therapy before relapse.

Survival was computed as the number of years from the date of gold-seed implantation to date of death due to any cause or to date of last follow-up evaluation for those patients still alive. The time to recurrence, or the disease-free interval, was computed as the number of years from gold-seed implantation to first recurrence.

Overall, 60 patients (44 percent) have remained clinically free of prostate cancer throughout the follow-up period or until death from other causes. Local progression developed in 39 percent of the patients and distant metastases in 42 percent. The chance of recurrence was clearly influenced by the stage and grade of the primary tumor as well as lymph node involvement.

Data showed that the estimated chance of death from prostate cancer at 15 years was 33 percent plus or minus 8 percent, and from all other causes, 72 percent plus or minus 8 percent. The presence of pelvic nodal metastases is the most powerful prognostic feature for recurrence of prostate cancer following radiotherapy.

Source: J. A. Eastham, M. W. Kattan, S. Groshen, P. T. Scardino, E. Rogers, C. E. Carlton, S. P. Lerner. Fifteen-year survival and recurrence rates after radiotherapy for localized prostate cancer. *Journal of Clinical Oncology* 15, 10 (1997):3214–3222.

ing an optimist with the new medical alternatives, I chose to believe that seed implants was the way to go. Also, one of the facilitators of our support group had seed implants and had survived 11 years—and he'd had the procedure when it was done by hand and not by ultrasound. He had no side effects from it, and he was healthy,

*Brachytherapy (seed implants).*  Brachytherapy uses radiation delivered from tiny radioactive "seeds" (stored in hollow wires) inserted directly into the prostate gland (interstitially) while the patient is under anesthesia. The seeds, either radioactive iodine 125 or palladium 103, are inserted below the scrotum under ultrasound guidance. They give off radiation continuously for a few weeks or months, depending on the type of seeds used. In almost all cases, the seeds are in place forever. For the most part, the radiation is contained in the prostate gland. However, during the first two months after the procedure, your doctor may ask you to take some precautions depending on the type of therapy you've received. For example, you may be instructed to wear a condom during sexual intercourse and avoid close prolonged contact with children or pregnant women. Your health care provider will give you specific instructions. Brachytherapy may be used in conjunction and/or combination with external beam radiation.

Advantages:
- Because seeds are placed at the site of the cancer, they can deliver more radiation directly to the prostate gland than can external beam radiation therapy.
- Apparently causes less long-term incontinence or impotence than with external-beam radiation or prostatectomy.
- May have quicker recovery time than radical prostatectomy.

Disadvantages:
- Requires surgical procedure to implant seeds and procedure cannot be repeated.
- Risks associated with anesthesia.
- Can irritate bladder and rectum.
- Can cause difficulty in urination, infection, diarrhea, or bleeding.
- Long term follow-up and results are lacking.
- Some medical centers add external-beam radiation to your treatment.

Cost: $15,000–$20,000; $22,000 if used with external radiation (1997 estimates).

Insurance coverage: Varies; check with your insurance carrier. Medicare has approved payment for brachytherapy, since it is considered a form of radiation, which has been covered for many years.

# Complementary Therapies

Many of you may already use complementary therapies or have heard of them. In fact, many of you will probably use some form of this therapy either alone or in conjunction with other more traditional treatments. If you do use complementary therapies, it's important that you tell your health care provider, because these therapies may affect how your traditional treatments are given or how they work. For example, alternative drugs, foods, or vitamins may increase the side effects of some medical therapies such as radiation, or even decrease its effectiveness.

Many of these agents have never been studied in well-controlled medical settings. Reports about their effectiveness are only anecdotal, that is, someone told someone else the product helped them. If you feel that one of more of these therapies is helping you, and it is not interfering with other treatments, then you may want to continue them. But remember, it is important that your medical team knows what you are taking or doing, because they will want to make sure there is no harmful interaction with your prescribed treatments. Before starting on any complementary therapy, you'll also want to check if your health insurance covers the cost.

Some examples of complementary therapies include:

- Acupuncture—a 2,000-year-old Chinese technique to relieve pain or cure disease by inserting fine needles into designated points on the body that relate to specific organs and body functions.
- Biofeedback—a training program designed to develop one's ability to control involuntary functions like heart rate, blood pressure, and skin temperature or to relax certain muscles. It is used successfully to help control incontinence.
- Chinese herbs—herbal preparations dating back to the ancient Chinese. Prescribed in complex formulas, Chinese herbs are believed to help restore balance in the body and help maintain a healthy inner peace. They can be provided in bulk form for tea, in granules or as tablets. PC SPES is the most popular of these herbs.
- Guided imagery—often used with relaxation techniques to try and help control feelings of pain, nausea, and tension. Patients are instructed to visualize a pleasant scene and relax into it. Audiotapes are sometimes useful.

*(continues)*

**Complementary Therapies** *(continued)*

- Herbal teas—Essiac tea, green teas; thought to have antioxidant activity.
- Hydrazine sulfate—drug said to help cancer patients maintain their appetite, nutrition, and weight. Some doctors say it helps avert the effects of cachexia, the wasting syndrome suffered by many cancer patients. Some patients claim it has stopped and reversed their cancer. However, two completed Phase III studies did not show this to be the case. The drug interacts with many other drugs such as antidepressants and should be used only with your doctor's knowledge.
- Low-fat, no-fat diets, macrobiotic diets—studies have suggested that there is a link between prostate cancer and diets high in red meats and animal fats; macrobiotic diets are low in fat and contain high amounts of brown rice, beans, whole grains, and seaweed.
- Meditation—the act of contemplative thinking. Transcendental meditation (TM) is a type of meditation based on ancient Hindu practices in which an individual tries to relax by repeating a mantra. The value of TM in treating various conditions is under investigation.
- Modified citrus pectin—modified form of a natural fruit fiber believed to make cancer cells too slick to stay in one place or clump together; in clinical trials.
- Ozone therapy—ozone or oxygen therapy comes in different forms: by direct infusion of ozone into the bloodstream or by diluting drinking water with hydrogen peroxide. The theory behind it is that hostile microorganisms and cancer cells cannot survive high oxygen concentrations. It's also believed that oxygen therapy restores the body's oxygen balance to a healthier level.
- Selenium—a metal found in the body. It acts as an antioxidant by protecting cell membranes from attack by free radicals. It also reacts with toxic metals such as mercury, cadmium, and arsenic to form biologically inert compounds. There is also a correlation between night vision and the selenium content of the retina; the higher the selenium content, the better the vision.

*(continues)*

**Complementary Therapies** *(continued)*

- Shark cartilage—used as a possible cancer treatment because of sharks' natural resistance to cancer. Bovine (cow) cartilage is also used in some preparations. It may prevent the development of blood vessels in solid tumors. It is currently in clinical studies in Canada and the United States.
- Soy foods—soy milk, tofu, tempeh, soybean curd; soy-based foods are believed to help block cancer-causing hormones from attaching to cell walls, thus stopping or slowing the growth of a tumor. Genistein, which is a chemical found in soybeans, is believed to also slow prostate tumor growth by acting like a female hormone.
- Vitamins A, C, E, selenium, and carotenes—antioxidants believed to help in the prevention of cancer by stopping free radicals from forming. Free radicals are high-energy, unstable chemical substances that cause cell damage that can lead to the development of cancer.
- Vitamin D—thought to inhibit cancer cell growth and enhance the immune system. The human prostate and prostate cancer cells contain vitamin D receptors. The best source of vitamin D is the sun. Sardines, tuna, and fortified milk are other good sources. Higher doses of vitamin D can cause hypercalcemia. Analogues of vitamin D that do not induce hypercalcemia have now been synthesized. Prescription vitamin D is much more powerful than ordinary vitamin D and should be discussed with your doctor.

functioning, and going strong. That helped me to make my decision to go that direction. I figured I wanted to be like him when I grow up."

If there is a common theme running through this chapter, it is that we are all highly motivated people. We have our fair share of self-confidence and self-esteem, and it affected how we approached our disease. As Charlie describes it, "People with high self-esteem are more likely to feel that they're not going to be knocked down. They're *not* just a bowling pin, and this big ball coming down the alley is *not* going to knock them over. I'm going to jump or skip or I'm going to hold my hand out and deflect it, but that devil's not going to knock me down. People like that are natural problem solvers, and having prostate cancer is just another challenge. That kind of attitude can exist in any background, in any individual," he argued, "and it can exist in any occupation."

Charlie always knew he wanted to be a lawyer when he grew up. "Intellectually, I just knew it was a calling," he remembers. "When I became a trial lawyer, there was a tremendous sense of bringing justice, particularly as an assistant state's attorney in Chicago. I put away a lot of bad guys, and that made me very happy. That's probably because I'm a very dominant individual—a results-oriented, self-confident, do-it-my-way, have-impact-on-the-world kind of guy. If I'm at a meeting or if I'm in an organization, things will happen. I took responsibility for my work, and I expected others to do the same. And this had a bearing on how I reacted to my diagnosis."

At that point, several of us wanted to know why, if he were so dominant and results-oriented, he abdicated his role in treatment decisions and deferred to his doctor—at least in the beginning. Charlie went on to explain, and it struck a familiar chord.

"When I was diagnosed, I immediately felt that I did not cause this—therefore, this was not my responsibility. The doctor was the expert on this. He's the guy with all the smarts, all the training. That's his job to fix it. It's going to cost a lot of money, no doubt, but the fact is that's why we pay you the big bucks. So I thought, 'I'm going to be okay,' and I had confidence that my doctor would fix it. So it wasn't really abdicating responsibility. It was simply, 'That's your job!' I delegated.

"So when I went to my urologist after being referred by my internist, I had two things going for me," Charlie continued. "One was total ignorance of the disease; the other was I had no fear. So when my urologist smiled at me as he talked about radical prostatectomies, I knew that was the choice of treatment he wanted me to have, and I said fine. I didn't think about cure or not cure. I didn't really think it was a serious deal. In fact, I thought I'd have the surgery and it would be over in two weeks. I was so stupid as I look back on it today. I can't believe that someone with my background and fundamental aggressiveness as a lawyer would ever go into a situation with that kind of response. Nevertheless, at that time, I did. Again, it wasn't until I talked with Lloyd Ney and PAACT that I really wised up, and that's where I did a 180-degree turn in every way. Unfortunately, I wasn't empowered before I made my decision to have a radical prostatectomy and radiation, and that has had—and continues to have—tremendous ramifications on my health."

Of all the stories we heard at the retreat, we were particularly blown away by Don's. Don's a soft-spoken man who packs a heck of a story. He even surprised us with some of his treatments and rituals, all delivered in his matter-of-fact, down-to-earth style.

"When I was first diagnosed, I asked the doctor, 'How long do I have?' He says, 'Well, probably a year or two at the most.' Then he asks, 'Radiation, radical, or chemo?' I said, 'We're going to wait on this a bit.' In the meantime, I'd heard about the organization PAACT and called Lloyd Ney. He gave me a lot of information on combination hormonal therapy. Now, I'm not used to using any drugs of any kind, any medication or anything, so hearing that I should go on this hormone therapy was really devastating, but after talking to Lloyd and getting encouragement from him, I had made up my mind to have it. I went back to my doctor, and I said I'd like to try CHT. So I started on the program of Lupron and flutamide."

However, that's not the end of the story. Don immediately began drawing on his practical experiences with animals and applied the information to himself.

"Being in the horse business for 38 years, shoeing horses, and working with the veterinarian profession, I see a lot of things that nutrition does for these animals," he went on to say. "So it made sense to me to consult a biochemist. My biochemist gave me tremendous hope. 'You can overcome this,' he said, and I believed him. Right away, I started working on my nutrition, my body chemistry, and a detoxification program to free my liver from toxins so I wouldn't have any problems with my liver. I came to understand that the medical people treat the symptoms and the nutritionist treats the cause. This is the theory behind the nutrition route. I've seen it in animals, particularly in animals infected with protozoa, which is a microorganism. The horses cannot function; they cannot jump. You put them on hydrogen peroxide and it kills the protozoa. It kills viruses. It kills everything. All of a sudden, the horse is functioning—he's back jumping, flexing, backbending, and back on the show circuit, when before he was useless, which was pretty much the way I felt. So I decided to try using hydrogen peroxide in my water, too. And hydrogen peroxide is a cheap medication, by the way—a gallon for $35 will last you a lifetime. I also use ozone therapy and ozone machines. They use this on race horses to oxygenate the body. You keep a lot of oxygen in the body with deep breathing; nutrition; and good, pure water. So, in other words, you treat the whole body rather than just the prostate. If I have a PSA of 2,448 and the doctors tell me it's going to be all over my body in a year—'Hey,' I thought, 'I'm going to treat everything!'"

So here you have ten men—ten very different men—embarking on different treatments and therapies. You can see that you have your work cut out for you, deciding what you're going to do. John had an observation that seemed to say it all: "We all are different in personality, but I think the one key here is that we're not afraid to eventually make a decision. There are a lot of people out there that just will not make a decision. They're like lemmings. They'll follow, and when they get to the cliff, they'll fall over the cliff. But we are all taking a different approach. You look at each and every one of us, and our personalities, our occupations, and where we live are so diverse that our chances of meeting like this would be next to nothing. But our one common key is perseverance. We perceive that we need to make a decision. We may take a year or two years to make it—we're detailers after all—but we make it."

A postscript: Keep in mind that these are all initial treatment decisions. Many of us had many more decisions ahead depending on how well our first line of defense worked. Nutrition took center stage as well, and most of us embarked on additional complementary therapies—all of which we'll explore in more detail later in the book.

With the blush of innocence quickly fading, we had all just begun.

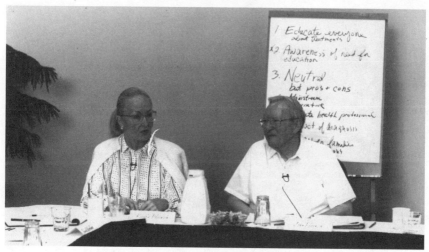

Rosalie and John Plosnich

# 3

# *Your Health Care Team*
## A PROACTIVE APPROACH

*I deal with the medical establishment on my terms. I'm empow-
ered. They're my consultants. I pay them.*
         *—Charlie Russ*

Empowerment. We use that term a lot and for good reason—being
empowered has changed our lives. It has become embedded in our
existence, and it is the essence of this book. For us, researching the
different treatment options revealed our need for knowledge, and
more knowledge on top of that, and gave us the confidence to begin
taking control.

How you select your health care providers demands scrutiny
equal to that of choosing a treatment. You'll want the most skilled
specialist you can find—someone who has performed your chosen
therapy countless times. Our first piece of advice is, don't settle for a
doctor by default or by quick referral unless you're completely comfortable with him or her. Second, as Lynne Zank quickly pointed
out, "Don't be intimidated by the doctors."

"They've got the technical skills," John added, "but we've been
through the school of hard knocks."

We all know that dealing with doctors can sometimes be a very
frustrating experience—not enough time, feelings of helplessness,
lack of control, and yes, intimidation. Have you ever heard of
"white coat hypertension"? For many people, just the sight of a
doctor's white lab coat is enough to raise their blood pressure. But it
doesn't have to be that way. Being empowered with your doctors
means taking a proactive role—asking questions and getting answers, combining their knowledge with yours, and using that

knowledge to make informed decisions. It's not a unilateral task. Your doctor also bears some responsibility in developing a good working relationship. In fact, he or she may need a healthy dose of humility.

"Sometimes I think that some members of the medical profession forget that people think," observed Manuel. "They tend to perceive that most people have no brains and are idiots who don't think for themselves."

"If you've got knowledge, then you're able to sit down and talk with your doctor," Bob added. "You're able to let him know that you can talk intelligently about the problem and that he's going to have to deal with you because you want certain answers. In fact, a knowledgeable, proactive approach with your doctor is the best way to get his attention."

Slowly but surely, doctors *are* beginning to pay attention. In fact, Rosalie Plosnich told us that doctors who lecture at the US TOO support groups are both surprised and impressed by the quality of the questions they get. "They're mind-boggled by the sophistication and intensity, the desire to know. They're amazed! They come in prepared to give a kindergarten-level speech, and they find out they're not only talking on a graduate level but they're talking bio-chemistry."

Don't panic! You don't have to be fluent in biochemistry to get your doctor's attention. Just let him or her know that you intend to be an active member of your health care team and wish to be treated as such.

So what exactly does this health care team consist of, and how do you pull one together? Well, that will depend partly on the stage of your disease, partly on your choice of treatment, and partly on personalities, both yours and those of your potential doctors. Remember, your health care team will become a very important part of your life, and you'll need people with whom you can work and with whom you are comfortable.

Sometimes, however, it's difficult knowing where and how to start. "One of the reasons I had trouble coming to any conclusions about what I wanted to do was because I didn't know any doctors," Derek recalled. "I'd been on the run, not settled anywhere, hadn't had a family doctor for years, since I retired in 1969. That's one of the reasons I started talking to everybody I could think of."

# Health Care Specialties

*Family Physician.*   A family physician is a primary care or other health care provider (e.g., nurse practitioner) who can treat all members of the family. If your family doctor or health care provider is concerned about the findings of a routine digital rectal exam (DRE) or PSA test, he or she will probably refer you to a urologist for further evaluation or a biopsy.

*Medical Oncologist.*   This health care provider has special training in the diagnosis, treatment, and evaluation of cancer and in the use of chemotherapy drugs and hormonal therapy to treat cancer. He or she has also had training in internal medicine. A medical oncologist can follow you concurrently with your urologist.

*Oncology Nurse.*   An oncology nurse specializes in the care of people with cancer. Oncology nurses take an active role in pain and symptom management.

*Radiation Oncologist.*   A radiation oncologist specializes in the use of radiation to treat cancer. Radiation may be used to treat early or advanced prostate cancer. A radiation oncologist can follow you concurrently with your urologist.

*Urologist.*   Urologists specialize in the diagnoses and treatment of diseases of the urinary tracts of men and women and the genital organs of men. They perform the surgeries for prostate cancer, including radical prostatectomies. Urologists may administer hormonal therapy and/or follow you concurrently with your oncologist.

Most of us were diagnosed by a urologist or immediately referred to one. "After John found out he had a PSA of 182," Rosalie told us, "the cardiologist told him he had to go to a urologist right away. Our cardiologist did not know enough about oncology to send us to a good medical oncologist who would be in the catbird seat as an objective neutral. He sent us to a surgeon who wanted to do surgery."

Most urologists perform surgery. However, if you choose to have a radical prostatectomy, you'll want to shop around for the "pro," as Bud put it. "The difference between the pros and peddlers is no different with doctors than it is in management out in the business field," he says. "The peddlers try to solve their own problems, and they don't solve anybody else's. The pros solve the other person's

---

## Questions to Ask Potential Health Care Providers

- Are they board certified in their specialty areas?
- How much experience have they had?
- How do they stay up-to-date on treatments?
- Do they participate in clinical studies?
- What hospitals and treatment centers do they work with?
- If you are undergoing surgery, how frequently does the surgeon perform the procedure?
- Are they comfortable with your seeking additional opinions?
- Do they accept your insurance?

## Questions to Ask Yourself

- Were you comfortable with this individual?
- Did you feel that he or she took enough time with you?
- Were your questions treated with respect and answered fully?

---

problems, and they automatically solve their own. In other words, the doctor that stays good at it doesn't have to worry about his income. He's going to build it up just fine. The fella that's out there to just jump in and do the first thing he has to fill his pocketbook—sooner or later it catches up to him."

In fact, a recent study of long-term survival rates in women with breast cancer indicated that those whose surgeries were done by the most skilled surgeons, that is, those who performed the surgery routinely versus those who did it only occasionally, survived longer. We assume this is also true of prostate cancer.

If you need surgery, it will be to your benefit to select a surgeon who does it frequently with few complications and with great success. It is also your right to ask the surgeon at the hospital for post-surgical infection rates and for a referral to other patients on whom he or she has operated. (Patient confidentiality has to be respected, however.) Talk to the hospital staff and find a way to talk to the operating room staff to see how they feel about a particular surgeon or staff physician. They can be a great source of information.

Sometimes just posing a few questions will tell you a lot about a prospective doctor. "I have to say that the original urologist Don consulted was not impressed with any of my questions or my being

---

*RT-PCR.* This is a blood test that can help determine whether the cancer has escaped the prostate gland. The test detects prostate cancer cells in the bloodstream. Currently, the test is not widely available.

---

there with Don," Lynne told us. "In fact, he was borderline rude. We tried to tell him some of the alternative things we were doing. He was a little interested at first because he's a runner—and we started to get encouraged—but then all of a sudden he said, 'Well, if you want to do native dancing, that's fine if you think it helps.' That was his attitude."

One thing to keep in mind is that most doctors receive no formal training in complementary or alternative medicine. They can't prescribe it, and they don't want to. And many say that their patients want only those solutions that are tried and true.

But if things don't seem quite right to you or your concerns aren't being addressed, tell your doctor how you feel. He or she may make every effort to address those concerns and rectify any problems. If not, don't be afraid to switch doctors. Trust and confidence are paramount to a successful partnership, and if you lose those, what have you got?

"It was interesting," Virgil remembers, "because the first urologist that I went to after being referred by my internist gave me an MRI and a CAT scan. In the course of talking to some people in the support groups on the Internet, they asked, "Did you do this test or that test?' I said no, and they asked why not. So I went back to my urologist and said, 'What about the RT-PCR?' He said, 'Well, I don't really believe in that.' I said, 'But Columbia developed it here in the urology department.' 'Yes,' he said, 'but I don't follow it.' So I said, 'What about the endorectal MRI?' He said, 'Well, some people believe in it, but I don't use it.' I said, 'I think I want to have it.' He said, 'I don't think you need it.' I said, 'Guess what? We're going to have it!' In fact—I fired him. I went and did the RT-PCR and the endorectal MRI, which really confirmed the presence of cancer and how far it had extended."

The underlying advice here is, if you feel strongly about an issue, don't be afraid to play a little verbal volleyball with your doctor, as Virgil and all of us have done.

## Understanding the Statistics

If your doctor recommends a specific treatment such as surgery, make sure he or she tells you about his or her personal experience with the procedure. For example, physicians may tell their patients that the rate of incontinence after a radical prostatectomy is only 10 percent—implying that that rate is the rate of incontinence for their patients. In reality, that particular doctor's percentage of patients who experience incontinence may be 40–50 percent. So make sure that your doctor is relating her experience and not quoting general statistics. You may also want to ask if it's possible to speak with any patients on whom she has performed the procedure. Patient confidentiality, however, must be respected.

As John pointed out, "You've got to start thinking in terms of yourself and not about hurting the doctor's feelings. You're the one who has to live with whatever decision he or she makes, and the more people you get involved in this thing, the so-called experts, the better. However, it does take courage to fire your urologist or any physician you are working with."

"You have to realize," Virgil continued, "that I've never been enamored with authority anyway, so I started talking to a lot of other urologists, and when it came down to the fact that I was going to have surgery, I then asked, 'Who's the best surgeon around here?' I went on the Internet to groups and had them give me names, and I narrowed it down to two doctors in New York. I went with Olsson and when I interviewed him, I had my questionnaire that I had set up in terms of all the things I wanted to find out. I said, 'Based on what you know about my case, what is your prognosis?' He said, 'Well, based on my last 900 procedures, this is what you can expect.' I said, '900?!' He said, 'Yeah, I've done 900 now since I've gotten better.' I said, 'This is the kind of guy I want to work with. I want a guy who knows what he's doing, does it regularly, and who's got good numbers behind him.'"

You want the "pro."

Charlie added his own two cents' worth on statistics. "The medical profession goes bonkers about statistics to justify what they're doing, and we should take note of how they think, how they approach treatments, and how they offer choices to patients. They tend to forget that each patient has a unique body and mind. They stick to conventional treatments and are always aware of possible malpractice actions."

Even if your urologist has "good numbers behind him" he still might not be a good match for you. Is your doctor a compassionate and caring individual? Is that important to you? If the status of your disease changes, will these traits be more or less important? These are personal questions that only you can answer.

When asked about the importance of sensitivity in doctors, Phyllis Georgeades shared some painful memories. "Paul is no longer in touch with his first urologist," she told us. "Paul would become very depressed every time he would have an appointment with him because he was like—if you could imagine an SS officer . . ."

At which point Rosalie bluntly visualized, "A cold, unfeeling fascist?"

"Exactly," Phyllis continued. "Every time Paul came out of the office, he would start sobbing. And he's a pretty tough guy. He would be so depressed and I said, 'Why are you going to him? What's he doing for you anyway? Your surgery's over.' I said, 'We need to find somebody else.' One of the last things Paul's sister told him before she died from cancer was, 'Find a good oncologist.' It so happened that during this period of time, he started attending a local support group and began to hear oncologists and urologists who would come and lecture. We went to about four oncologists before Paul found the one he likes and is comfortable with. And now he comes away and feels so great. Of course, he's more educated in all the other aspects of the treatment, too. Maybe it was the education that made him feel better, but I know the first urologist was not helping him emotionally. He may have done wonderful work—the mechanical skills were there—but the bedside manner was not."

For some men, bedside manner isn't an issue as long as the technical skills are there. Again, it's a highly personal choice. You need to decide whom you're most comfortable with and who inspires the most trust.

As Bob put it, "One of the things we haven't addressed is that, fine, we know that a lot of doctors aren't good communicators and can be very insensitive, but if you have a choice between a real good mechanic and one who isn't a good mechanic but has a good flow of words, which one are you going to choose? I want the good mechanic working on me, and I don't care how he talks!"

Of course, you're more than an inanimate pile of parts, so you might want to try to find a balance between skill and compassion—with all your doctors. Usually, a urologist will be the first member of your team. But depending on the stage of your disease, you may switch to an oncologist or work with both specialists.

"I really don't formally see a urologist anymore, but I have a continuing relationship with one," Peter told us. "I see him at support group meetings and periodically make an appointment just to talk with him, sort of let him know what's new with me and find out what's new with him. In my mind, he's a member of my team, even though I'm not using him currently for treatment, because I'm under the care of an oncologist."

"Here's how I see the different philosophies," Manuel explained. "An oncologist is primarily and exclusively concerned with getting rid of the cancer. He doesn't particularly care about issues like nerve-sparing. He wants to get the cancer out, period. That's it. As a matter of fact, they are afraid that some cells may be there, so that's what they want to get rid of. Now, a good urologist sees it with certain quality-of-life issues. They're concerned with incontinence and impotence and will do whatever needs to be done even though you may compromise the cancer progression."

To be fair, a *good* oncologist will also be concerned with your quality of life and will factor your values and wishes into any treatment decision. He or she will consult you for your opinion—just as you are consulting your doctor. Don't forget to tap into the skill and knowledge of an oncology nurse if one is available. Oncology nurses are highly trained professionals who can be particularly helpful with symptom management and pain management—if that's an issue for you.

There are many other factors that will influence your selection of doctors. Obviously, one factor is location and the time and money you're willing to invest in the selection process. Most of us consulted several doctors from many different institutions. Derek, as you'll recall, crisscrossed the country looking for doctors who satisfied his need for excellence and competence.

"In my case," Derek explained, "I empowered myself to say, 'I'm not going to take the advice of you or you or you because you haven't satisfied me yet.' To hear people say, 'You have to believe in the doctor, no matter what'—I can't do that."

"I was fortunate to travel from my hometown down to Sarasota, Florida, and meet two great doctors," Bud remembers. "They were so far ahead of other areas that it made the difference in maybe saving my life. I went home four months later and had a terrible time finding a urologist who would give me a shot of Lupron or give me a prescription for Eulexin. They didn't want to even talk about it. This is what really turned me off. Then when I heard about some of the new things that were being done, I said to one of my doctors, 'Here's a great thing they're doing.' He would reply, 'Oh, we did that 20 years ago in school.' And I said, 'But doc, you didn't have the same equipment to do it.' He just shut me off, and that's what bothers me. I know they have to be sure before they use it, that it's going to work, but some of them have tunnel vision and they just don't want to accept change. The greatest thing we have to have in this life is a reason to accept change, and when the scientific medicine becomes great medicine, it becomes an art. Those artists are the doctors who stay on top of it and do the best they can."

"The problem with cryotherapy," Derek explained, "is that many doctors aren't being trained to perform it properly. They're not checking to make sure the freezing is accurate and complete. I feel it's a great procedure if it's done properly. There are over 200 hospitals out there using it, but I can't say there are 200 hospitals doing a good job."

"I think that's true of any procedure," Virgil commented.

"That's exactly what I'm saying," replied Derek. "It's the individual doctor performing the procedure. To give cryotherapy a bad name because it's not successful isn't a fair shake because there are a lot of doctors out there who do a good job at it. Just like surgeons. There are good surgeons out there. You've got one. I know of good ones in Albuquerque."

Good doctors, we all agreed, immediately refer their patients to support groups, too. "It's so important that we get the doctors to cooperate with us on this issue," Derek passionately explained. "Our support group in Albuquerque decided to get the names of all the urologists in town and split them up into groups for interviews. I had a group from one hospital and simply went to the hospital, gave them my card, and said, 'Here's who I am and I would like to interview your doctors.' Not all of them will talk to you. Not all of them want you talking to their patients. In fact, my group of doctors

In August 1996, the AUA recognized cryotherapy as no longer investigational or experimental. This was the result of a PAACT initiative driven by Charlie Russ and resolved with the considerable help of Dr. Charles McKeil, a cryourologist and then president of the AUA.

stopped talking to me because I was asking questions that put them on the spot. And it's interesting. I would get different answers from different surgeons because each did things differently. But the good ones are going to start sending their patients to support groups. Those are the doctors who are really honest and doing a good job and don't mind being scrutinized. Then we can start talking to these cancer patients and really start educating them. They'll learn that it's OK to be proactive. It's OK to ask questions. And that, ultimately, benefits both the doctor and the patient."

"If you don't ask questions," Bob added, "you can make a wrong decision that will alter your life forever. I've heard some men say, 'Well, the doctor knows what he's doing. I'll take his word for it.' It's not *his* life. It's not *his* decision to make. He can only tell you things and advise you. *You* are in charge of your life. You make the final decisions. If he makes the decision, he can render you hopelessly and helplessly altered for the rest of your life."

We talk from experience. Many of us, including John, Peter, and Charlie, were initially misdiagnosed, which delayed crucial treatment. So if we seem a bit harsh in our assessments, we mean to be—because we don't want you making the same mistakes we did. We're just saying, be informed.

Charlie's views of the medical profession became apparent during our first discussion period, particularly with regard to the American Urological Association. At the time, the AUA's position on cryotherapy was firm: It was investigational and experimental. In fact, according to Charlie, many urologists simply didn't tell their patients about this option, instead stressing the need for a radical prostatectomy.

"I would take the whole AUA and reorganize it if I could," Charlie passionately stated. "I would sue many of the doctors for malpractice if I could." Manuel instantly perceived this as intense anger boiling over, but Charlie begged to differ. "It's not anger, really," he said. "I'm actually really cool about it. It would just be a matter of simple justice."

"There's a heavy rejection in here of doctors by all of us," Charlie later observed. "By rejection, I mean being skeptical. Not taking them as God, not accepting them as being the overall final purpose and source of wisdom, and taking the responsibility to help cure ourselves."

That, however, is a big responsibility, and you may or may not feel comfortable calling the shots. In fact, you probably won't—at least at first—and that's OK, too. That's why it's important that you become a team player *with* your doctor. You work together to optimize your care. It's something we all actually agreed on and something Manuel wanted to emphasize. "I have a little problem with what I consider radicalism," he said. "I see in some of us a tendency to be radical. I am a person of the middle way, maybe because I am an Episcopalian. I think the doctor went to school for many, many years and trained very hard, and I have to recognize that. He's trained in the medical field the same way that a lawyer is trained in that field. I don't think that I have the knowledge that it takes to decide something on law, because I don't have that training. There's got to be some middle ground."

Peter reiterated the point Charlie was trying to make earlier. "Most of us are not rejecting the medical community. We're changing them from being God figures to being consultants."

"We want to find out—how can this doctor help me?" Paul added. "What can he do? We should try to do those things that are going to be the most beneficial to us, but I believe that we shouldn't really challenge him, as Charlie put it. Certainly we can make our own judgments and choices and all those things, but when we go in there, why get into an argument? I'm trying to say, we need to suck up as much of his brain information as we can and get all the benefits we can. And the trick is, how can we do this most effectively?"

"I don't take them on as a challenge," Charlie responded, "and I don't get into arguments with them. I do take them on as team members. When I go to my doctors, I tell them, "Look, let me explain to you what I am. I am an empowered patient, and this means that I consider you my consultant. I consider you my partner. I consider that you are someone who is going to join me in a search for answers. I'm going to keep a lot of questions on a computer, and I'm going to come to our meetings with a computer report. I'll give you a copy. I'll ask a lot of questions of you, but I'll also supply you with a lot of information and documentation to back up what I'm saying. If I see something of interest, I'll bring it with me. Maybe it's something you've read; maybe it's something you haven't read. It's a continuing education session for both of us.'"

"Exactly," Paul concluded. "It's a sharing of information. If you have to yell at them, swear at them, fine. Whatever it takes to get the information out. Or—take them a box of candy."

So basically, what we're saying is that education becomes a two-way street. You get information from your doctor, your support group, your library, or wherever you can. Your doctor can also get information and suggestions from you.

"We've got to realize," John reminded us, "that technology is moving so rapidly in all fields, that eventually these fellas have tunnel vision because they don't really know what's out there. Anytime I get information, some of it will go to my doctors because there are things here that have to be explored. But if you don't bring this information to the good doctor, you're not going to have this opportunity."

Charlie gave us an illustration. "When I got my first bone scan results, I said to my doctor, 'Listen, you didn't count the foci,' and he said, 'What?' I said, 'You didn't count the foci.' He said, 'Why is that important?' I said, 'Because Dr. Bob Liebowitz, who is on the board of PAACT, believes that's a good indication of the aggressiveness of the cancer and here's his statement on it.' So he took that, and I said, 'By the way, I noticed on my blood test that I'm not getting a liver enzyme test.' He looked sheepishly at me and said, 'Oh yes, I forgot that.' So this is how you help educate your doctor."

By now, you may be saying that this is all fine and dandy, but you're in a managed-care plan or HMO and time and dollars are at a premium. In all fairness, many doctors these days are under very tight time constraints, often obligated to see a certain number of patients per hour. So you may have only a very small window of opportunity to get your questions answered. However, as John says, "My time is just as valuable as his time, and if he can't take an extra five or ten minutes to answer my questions, whether it's yes or no or in more detail, I'll go to another doctor."

In order to alleviate the time crunch, many doctors are making use of multimedia educational tools. Bud told us of a couple of doctors he knows who are using videos to help educate their patients. "I think

## The Patient's Bill of Rights

A movement toward patient empowerment was started in the early 1970s when the American Hospital Association developed the Patient's Bill of Rights. This document has become the standard for the health care industry. It may be helpful for you to keep these rights in mind throughout your experience with cancer and cancer treatments.

1. The patient has a right to considerate and respectful care.
2. The patient has a right to obtain from his or her physician complete current information about his or her diagnosis.
3. The patient has a right to obtain from his or her physician information necessary to give informed consent prior to the start of any procedure and/or treatment.
4. The patient has the right to refuse treatment to the extent permitted by law.
5. The patient has a right to every consideration of his or her privacy concerning his or her own medical care program.
6. The patient has a right to expect that all communications and records pertaining to his or her care should be treated as confidential.
7. The patient has a right to expect that within its capacity a hospital must make reasonable response to the request of a patient for services.
8. The patient has a right to obtain information as to any relationship of his or her hospital to other healthcare and educational institutions insofar as his or her care is concerned.
9. The patient has a right to be advised if the hospital proposes to engage in human experimentation affecting his or her care and the right to refuse to participate in such research projects.
10. The patient has the right to expect reasonable continuity of care.
11. The patient has the right to examine and receive an explanation of his or her bill regardless of the source of payment.
12. The patient has the right to know what hospital rules and regulations apply to his or her conduct as a patient.

---

### Informed Consent

It's your doctor's responsibility to provide you with enough information about your treatment options so that you can make an informed choice. Your doctor should explain exactly

- what treatment options are recommended,
- what the likely effects are (both good and bad),
- why it is being done,
- the expected outcome with or without treatment,
- your alternatives to receiving a particular treatment.

---

this is great," he says. "Some doctors have a 15-minute tape they hand to their patients and say, 'Go into my room here and listen to it. This tells you the six different options that you have. In fact, you don't have to look at it today. You can take it home and be comfortable. I want to be your doctor, but I want you to decide what is the best of these treatments.' This doctor wrote to me and said, 'I was talking to a couple of my friends, and we agreed that we just don't have enough time. We're so busy. People can tell us we're terrible doctors and all, but we're on a patient schedule, and if we're 20 minutes late and you're the next guy coming in, you're going to cuss us down. And yet if we do everything that you people out there want, we can't do it.' So now they give out these tapes. One doctor had hundreds of them made. He says, 'Take this home, look at it, then come back in a week and we'll discuss it.' I'm telling you this just to let you know that we're really making headway on this problem."

Again, as John reminded us, "there are a lot of good doctors around. We don't want to lose sight of that because doctors do play an important part in our lives."

"Just remember that doctors are not infallible," Manuel concluded. "No one is. When you're diagnosed with prostate cancer, you have to go through a certain progression of events. And it's not simple. In many cases, you just don't know if the cancer has spread. It's like exploring the universe. We're now finding planets and solar systems that have been there all along. We just didn't know that they existed. You may be given good news—your cancer has been caught early, you have many options—and you may strike it lucky with the option that you choose or you may not."

One of those options is complementary, alternative, or unconventional medicine and consulting alternative health care providers. Whatever you call it, complementary therapy can be a valuable addition to your health care agenda. It certainly was—and continues to be—for most of us.

"Much of my whole experience has been unconventional," Virgil told us. "For a very long time, I have believed in alternative therapies. When I came out of 'Nam, I gained a greater appreciation for the Asian culture. I understood a big difference in the way they lived their lives and the way they could see life compared to a Western way of civilization. I was fortunate enough to be able to work for some companies that gave me the opportunity to travel around the world, and I saw other cultures, a lot of Asian culture especially, and it started me thinking about what I could learn from this, what it could bring to my existence that could create a better way. So I got into a lot of the martial arts, and I got into meditation, into visualization, into doing the things that seemed to me to be more natural and healthier.

"So when I got my diagnosis, when I first got the PSA, I kind of knew at that point I had cancer," Virgil continued. "I just figured that there was a lot of evidence out there that suggested I probably had it. So I said, 'OK, what are we going to do about it? How are we going to deal with it?' Immediately, I interviewed all the doctors, and they went through all their tests. In other words, I went the traditional route. But I also went the alternate route simultaneously. I went to my acupuncturist, who called in a specialist from China. Their examination of me was very interesting. They looked at my tongue, they looked underneath my tongue, they looked in my eyes, they checked my pulse, they touched my toes. They conferred and started a program of herbal teas and acupuncture to prepare me for the surgery. They said, 'We cannot cure cancer. There's nothing we can do that's going to stop the cancer or necessarily retard it. We think you should have the surgery and remove it, but then once it's done, we've got other things we're going to do to bring you back.' So at that point, it was a wonderful experience from all the others I had—15 guys crawling up my butt as opposed to this very civilized, holistic kind of approach."

Don, as you'll recall, was also looking for a holistic approach—a way to treat his whole body as opposed to one part. That's why he consulted and hired a biochemist. "My biochemist didn't really have any contact with the medical community," Don remembers. "He had been a cancer patient himself; he'd been burned with radiation and has problems with his voice. But he's been in this field for years and years. It's almost like an underground system as far as I'm concerned. Anyway, we started working immediately on my biochemistry, my body pH, the detoxification program, and I changed my diet, drastically. And I have to say my wife, Lynne, was 100 percent behind me. She's the backbone behind all this."

"I pretty much let him do what he felt he needed to do," responded Lynne. "I did have an appointment with the nutrition therapist that I've gone to for a long time. Don didn't really want to go, but we talked about it a lot and he finally agreed to go. He was very tired, slept in the backseat all the way, went in kind of grudgingly, and came out a changed person from that time on. From that time on, Don became very gung ho, very interested in reading and researching alternative ways of handling this. He came out with hope."

Paul offered a postscript. "We have to appreciate that every one of us is different; every doctor is different. There are all these different procedures and approaches. None of us is 100 percent right. The doctors aren't always right. Nobody can make definite statements. That's why we have to be very careful. Especially when we're in support groups and we're presenting information. We should always be broad-minded and remember that your health care and all the decisions that you make are an individual and very personal thing."

# 4

# *Treatments*

## ACTION AND RECOVERY

*I felt that the day I had my surgery was a new birthday for me. I
was born again. I was given a second chance at life.*
—**Virgil Simons**

It was time. The options had been reviewed, the decisions were
made, and treatments were scheduled. The only thing left—just do
it.

Just do it! Surgery, seeds, ice, hormones, herbs, and ozone! We
were all preparing ourselves to undergo different treatments in different ways. (See Table 4.1 at the end of the chapter for a summary
of our diagnoses and treatments.)

"One of the first things I did for myself," Virgil remembers, "I decided to buy a new car before the surgery, which drove my wife
crazy. She didn't understand why I would want a new car. So I said,
'Hey, if nothing else, when you go to the funeral, you'll have a new
car to drive.'"

Dark humor aside, a little indulgence never hurts. In reality, Virgil
prepared for a radical prostatectomy in a much more practical way.

"After I gave the last unit of blood for my surgery," he recalled, "I
temporarily walked away from Western medicine. I said to myself,
'OK, now I'm going to go to the Eastern form and prepare myself.' I
created a mental picture of my prostate, and I visualized the cancer
inside of it. I visualized it getting smaller as I compressed it with my
energy to make certain it wasn't going to go anywhere. I live in New
Jersey, and the hospital where I was to have surgery is in New York,
and there's a point along the Hudson River where I could sit and
look across the river at the hospital. So I also visualized going into

the hospital—so I could be there the next morning, looking out for myself when I was unconscious in surgery."

"Visualization gave me tremendous strength. I began to feel in control of the situation. I began to feel I was taking back my life. You just let your mind go, and you can use visualization anywhere. I was doing it in the subway, at home, wherever and whenever I had some free time or when thoughts of what I was facing began to take over."

"I was visualizing on the tennis court," Bud jumped in. "Boy, did I visualize! Every time I was in a tennis tournament or a league game, every time I hit a tennis ball, I said, 'Take that, you little cancer sucker!' I hadn't thought of that till just now. And all these things make such a difference. There's a lot about this that doctors can't cure or even treat, but maybe we can help treat and cure ourselves."

"Exactly," Virgil continued. "So the morning of the surgery I was out of bed at 4:00 A.M. I had to be there at 6:30 in the morning. I was ready. I hopped on the gurney and said, 'Let's do it.' I really had no fear. I somehow knew I was going to come through this and be OK. And I was. One of the best things was the pain-management system. Whenever I felt bad and had a need for pain medication, I pressed this button and gave myself a little hit, and it wasn't bad. There really wasn't a lot of pain.

"I also had decided that I would take care of myself," Virgil continued. "I hired a nurse to come in at night to take care of me, just to give the responsibility over to somebody else—not because I didn't trust the capability of the hospital, but I knew that with budget cuts at night the staff's going to be cut. I didn't want to risk anything, and I didn't want to be subject to governmental influences. I was going to take care of myself. That was so important to me. The only thing I felt really bad about was the catheter. That was an intrusion!"

"That didn't bother me that much, the catheter," Manuel remarked. "I was used to seeing them in the hospice where I volunteered. I was terrified because I knew I was going to have one, but when I actually had it in, I just accepted it. I thought it would be extremely painful, and it wasn't. I wasn't even really aware it was in. In fact, I kind of saw it as a friend because it had a function. As far as the radical prostatectomy itself, I had no problems either. I recovered quickly."

So did Virgil. "My private nurse, Winston, was a great guy and probably helped my recovery tremendously in that he was kind of an extension of the same feelings I had—a very spiritual kind of person and very capable. So the first night, he said, 'You've got to get up out of bed. You're going to sit in the chair and I'm going to change the bed, get you washed up a little bit, and then we're going to take a walk.' So that's when the process of doing the night walks began, to get my insides moving again. So we walked and a couple of other guys joined us, and at that point the whole thing kind of crystallized in my mind. I knew immediately that I had beat it. The pathology report was irrelevant because I knew the cancer was gone. The report came back negative margins, negative vesicles, negative everything, and my PSA had dropped to less than 0.1. From that point, it was a matter of continually working to get back into strong physical shape. The biggest problem I had was the anesthesia, just getting the anesthesia out of my body, because that was really debilitating. Everything is physically shut down, and you're trying to get all the parts working again. I could feel the parts of my body struggling, trying to come back to normal. The second day, I told the nurses to take the pain-management system away, I could cut it out. I didn't really need it at that point. They said, 'Are you sure?' I said, 'Yeah, I'm sure.' The pain was going to be irrelevant. That was a help. I just started walking more, every chance I got. Getting out of bed the first couple of days hurt a little bit—pulling from the stitches—but I was going to do it. I was going to beat it."

Virgil delved a little deeper—actually much deeper—into his post-surgical promenades, giving us all a few laughs along the way: "The biggest epiphany came one morning early, about 3:00 A.M. when we were walking the halls of the hospital. I finally ripped off this fart, which was the best thing that could ever happen. You see, in terms of recovery, if you pass gas, they start giving you a liquid diet. You have a bowel movement, they give you solid food. So there's a prize at the bottom of the Cracker Jack box. So pass gas—give me that Jell-O! It was wonderful! The next carrot was to have a bowel movement because then I would get to go home, and I wanted to get out of there in the worst way. I had gone in Wednesday for surgery. Friday comes, still nothing, and I'm going crazy. I'm walking the halls like I'm preparing for a marathon. Fortunately, by Saturday, the wisdom of my doctor prevailed and he let me go home. He took the staples out, and I shuffled out the door with my catheter—my 'friend.'"

A postscript: "On Monday morning, I finally had my first bowel movement, which was, indeed, memorable. Nobody told me how bad this was going to hurt. But you talk about something setting you free. It was one of those things that hurt so good because it was just another hurdle to get past."

Unfortunately, not all of us breezed through surgery. In fact, for some of us the outcome was radically different.

"It wracked me up physically," Charlie told us. "The recovery process was long and hard. It took me a full year to recover from the radical prostatectomy. I remember coming out of the recovery room, and the doctor told me that the disease had escaped the capsule. At the time I didn't really understand the seriousness of that and so I didn't think much of it. Besides, my PSA went way down after the surgery. But then it started to slowly climb. When it reached 1.3, my doctor said, 'I think you ought to have radiation.' I said, 'Radiation?' He said, 'Yes, I think you ought to have it.' I had heard a lot of bad things about radiation, but I decided to go ahead with it because, again, I had complete faith in my doctor. They're part of America—apple pie, the flag, everything. So I went through seven weeks of radiation, which was painless. I had a very good radiation oncologist, and my PSA dropped down to 0.2. But radiation weakens you. It's very slow. It's very subtle. It's not devastating, but you do begin to feel tired after seven weeks of treatment. So you can see how I was 'answering the ad.' I was getting all the mainstream treatments, one after the other, until I started to bleed internally. I thought it was hemorrhoids. It went on and on until one night my wife took me to the emergency room and my hemoglobin was 7— normal hemoglobin is 15. I had lost over half my blood! It was very pleasant in the emergency room, quiet, peaceful. It was warm, and I thought, 'I'm going to enter another world, without a care of any kind.' The doctors were terrific. They stopped the bleeding, and I was admitted to the hospital. At that point, one doctor said, 'I'm going to fix you.' He took me into this room with these hyperbaric chambers. They slid me into one, which looked like a torpedo tube cut in half with a plastic top. Then, they actually turn these wheels, you know the wheels they turn in the movies, and half the guys are locked into the submarine and they all drown. Anyway, I go in there, a little uneasily. I don't have claustrophobia, but it's a good place to get it. I got pure oxygen for over an hour each day, five days a week for seven weeks. Pressurewise, they lower you 40 feet below sea level and pump pure oxygen into you—which really pumped me up. So that was another milestone in my treatment. Everything was fine. The bleeding stopped. My PSA was low. But all of a sudden, in June of 1994, my PSA jumped from 0.2 to 0.6.

"By this time I was a real graduate of the Hard Knocks University and getting empowered by the minute, and so I knew what was going on. I had already fired my urologist. I believe I never should have had the first TUR, and I never should have had the radical prostatectomy or the radiation. I should have been examined immediately for possible systemic cancer. Now, of course, my disease was systemic. My new urologist told me that I should try watchful waiting because he couldn't stage it. A second opinion at M.D. Anderson was the same. So here I am faced with the weight of the world of the medical profession and I say, 'OK, I'll try this for a little while.' But I started thinking that it was idiotic that they couldn't stage my disease and that it was probably even more idiotic to just watch and wait. That Christmas my doctors finally staged my disease at D2 because it had metastasized. So I told my oncologist that I was going on dual hormonal therapy immediately. I did that and my PSA shot down to zip and at the time my bone scans were still negative. However, in 1995 my PSA started rising again. I had become hormone refractory, and in June of that year the metastasis showed clearly on my bone scans. There was one foci, or spot on my ribs, and I have a tumor growing on my right pelvic bone. As of today, my PSA is 3.3. That's relatively low, but it's not my PSA that I have to worry about. It's the metastasis. Right now, I'm looking at all my options. I may go on Nizoral. I'm heavily into nutrition and PC SPES [Chinese herbs], and I'm considering clinical trials in immune therapy. I do have options."

It's pretty obvious that most of us do not have a lot of good things to say about radiation. But remember, these are our opinions and our personal experience talking. We won't sugarcoat what we've been through or deny our responsibility for our treatments.

"The radiation was the thing that really created a problem with me because I had a tremendous amount of damage," John told us. "Six weeks after my surgery to remove the tumor I received 37 radiation treatments, followed by 13 more in 1995 to help relieve back pain. I was on Coumadin for my heart condition, which is a blood thinner, and I was going along fine until I started to hemorrhage. And the bleeding didn't start until eight or ten months after the radiation treatments. You talk about hemorrhaging. I bled from my eyes, nose, mouth, and my ears; you name it. I was passing clots, getting plugged up, and when I went to the bathroom everything was red. Doesn't take much blood to turn water to red. So that's a bit of a shock to see all this blood."

"Nobody told us that when you radiate an area where there's been prior surgery that there's a potential problem," Rosalie interjected. "He'd had a hemorrhoidectomy and two hernia repairs. They radiated this section, and it turned all those adhesions and scar tissue into a bleeding pulp, and then when you give that patient Coumadin on top of it, there was no way he wasn't going to hemorrhage on it. This was clearly a case of medical mismanagement where he was being treated by one physician for one thing and another physician for another. They never communicated with each other to ensure that their respective treatments wouldn't be disastrous for John."

"I may start bleeding again," John added. "I don't know. A friend of my wife's asked, 'Have you tried cranberry juice?' I said, 'No, what's cranberry juice got to do with it?' She said, 'Well, my doctor recommended cranberry juice because it helps clear the system.' I said, 'Well, I'm not a woman, but by golly I'll try cranberry juice.' Since I've been taking it, I haven't bled! Besides, I like cranberry juice.

"I also had trouble swallowing because of the radiation," John told us. "That continued for almost a month before they gave me pills, and this was supposed to relieve it. Well, it didn't. I even had a problem swallowing water. Eventually, it started wearing off and I'm now back to normal."

Not so fast, John. There's something that hasn't worn off. Even after several years, Rosalie's disappointment with the medical establishment was apparent. "First of all, when he started the radiation treatments, they gave him no handbook, no counseling. They gave me no recipes, diets, suggestions, or anything. And radiation suppressed John's immune system, terribly. They had to butterfly his chest during the bypass surgery, and they had to open up the good leg that doesn't have phlebitis in it and take five grafts from his leg. The leg they took the grafts from ended up with a long, wide, and deep wound. It's the kind that has to be healed from the inside, so I had to take him at least once a week to have the surgeon dress the wound. The cardiac surgeon was very upset by the amount of time the wound was taking to heal, because the whole body system was suppressed by the radiation. When the rectal bleeding started, we found a good gastroenterologist and they started doing cauterization."

"I was a guinea pig," concluded John. "We're all guinea pigs. The radiation really didn't do anything for me. I was never able to get my PSA below 1. But I'm not incontinent. I don't wear a bag, and I'm very thankful for that. I make a lot of pit stops, but I'm also on diuretics for my heart. And here's some advice, and I've said this before—you have to ask your doctor questions. One question people just don't seem to ask a doctor is 'What are the aftereffects of this treatment?' Am I going to be not only impotent but have bleeding problems? Am I going to be incontinent and have to have a bag on the side of my leg that has to be emptied on a regular basis? Am I going to have infection in the area because the acidity of the urine is creating a problem? These are all factors that each and every one of us has to deal with. But if you don't ask those questions, your doctor probably won't automatically give you the information."

"Speaking of guinea pigs, my doctors told me, 'You're probably the guinea pig we're looking for,'" Bud remembers. "The FDA had just approved a new drug called Eulexin, and my doctors put me on it that day. Being an old reconnaissance man, I spent three hours in the library with my wife until we found some information on Eulexin. The research materials said that the drug stays in your bloodstream for 7.2 to 9.1 hours. I had been told to take it at mealtimes, and I said to my wife, 'This is ridiculous. I'm taking it at 8:00 in the morning, noon, and 6:00 at night. By 1:00 or 3:00 in the morning, these cancer cells are eating me up.' She looked at me and said, 'So what are you going to do about it?' I said, 'I'm going to call my doctor and tell him they're giving the medication wrong.' This is the honest truth and it's all been documented. Well, I called my doctor and he said, 'That's fine. We don't really object to you taking it every eight hours if that's what you want to do. Since we didn't know what effect it would have on an empty stomach, we thought that taking it with meals would be better.' So I said, 'I'll take it at 7:00 in the morning, 3:00 in the afternoon and 11:00 at night.' And I did that, and I did it every day, and I never forgot it. At the end of three months, my PSA was down to 3.3; my prostate was down to

> The half-life of Eulexin® in the body is 7.2 to 9.1 hours. Thus the drug would not have been completely gone, but in the middle of the night it could end up in less than ideal concentrations if not taken every eight hours.

almost normal size—about 15 grams. I was having no problems, and I was urinating normally.

"At the end of four months, my PSA was almost undetectable and my prostate was down to normal," Bud told us. "My doctor said he'd never seen such a dramatic recovery in a patient before. He wasn't sure what to advise me regarding radiation or surgery but that he would follow me closely with exams and bloodwork every three months. Then, at the first sign of any local recurrence, we could consider radiation or surgery.

"Well, I walked outside on cloud 9," Bud remembered with a smile. "My wife was waiting in the car. She asked, 'So what are you going to have, radiation or surgery?' I said, 'I'm not going to have anything.' She couldn't believe that my cancer was gone. So we marched back into the medical office, and my doctor told my wife that I had no signs of cancer. In fact, my doctor wrote in his monthly medical report that he'd never seen such a dramatic recovery in response to hormonal therapy.

"To make a long story short, I also talked to the VP of the pharmaceutical company that makes Eulexin and told him how I took the drug and about my recovery. He called me back a few days later and said, 'I've got good news for you.' I asked, 'What is it? Are you going to pay for my medicine?' And he says, 'No, I've got better news than that. We just sent out 25,000 letters this morning to every pharmacist in the United States and to every urologist in the United States and Canada and said it's important for patients to take this product every eight hours.'

"I continued taking the drugs for two more years and that kept my PSA down to zero. At that point, I asked my doctor how long I'd have to keep taking them, and he said probably the rest of my life. However, I decided to go off Eulexin because I had read that if you take it too long it can affect your liver. My doctor advised me not to stop the drugs, but I told him I was willing to still be the guinea pig. I'd stay on the Lupron, go off the Eulexin, and see what happened.

---

### Intermittent Hormonal Therapy (IHT)

Usually, combined hormonal therapy (CHT) will eventually stop working, and your PSA level will begin to rise. How fast this happens depends on how quickly hormone-resistant cancer cells grow and multiply in your body. CHT can also cause many unpleasant side effects such as hot flashes and a loss of sexual function. Long-term use can cause decreased muscle mass, bone loss, and liver damage. Because of these problems, some patients and their doctors choose to stop CHT for a time and carefully monitor PSA levels. If your PSA begins to rise, CHT can be started again, and the cycle can be repeated. This is called intermittent hormonal therapy, or IHT. IHT is still experimental, so if you're interested, talk over the benefits and risks with your doctor. What you value most and the quality of your life will also play a role in your decision. (A large national study is currently under way comparing CHT to IHT.)

Advantages:
- When you go off the therapy, you'll slowly return to the level of sexual function you were at just before beginning CHT. Other side effects such as hot flashes will go away or become less noticeable.
- Less expensive.
- IHT may extend the length of time that CHT therapy works.

Disadvantages:
- The main risk associated with intermittent therapy is that the disease may progress while you're not receiving treatment.

Cost: Varies with length and frequency of treatment cycles.

Insurance coverage: Yes.

---

"At the end of the year, my PSA was still down. So I went off Lupron as well. I was off both drugs for about a year, but unfortunately, my PSA went back up to 13.5. So my doctor put me back on both Lupron and Eulexin immediately. After three months the PSA was back to 1.1. But I was having hot flashes and my breasts were enlarging, so I decided to stop it again!

"Since then I've been on and off the drugs for about five years. People ask me, 'Why did you go off them?' I felt that this was

## When Hormonal Therapy Fails

When prostate cancer grows or causes problems despite the use of hormones, you still have many other options. This includes stopping hormonal therapy or antiandrogen therapy and undergoing radiation or chemotherapy. You may also want to consider trying new and unique therapies—some of which are under investigation.

Standard chemotherapy, although an option, has not been proven to be highly effective in advanced prostate cancer, and there are side effects from the drugs to consider. However, depending on your circumstances, you and your doctor may decide that chemotherapy is the best treatment for you at the time, and it may help relieve disease symptoms such as pain. Also, keep in mind that new drugs and new combinations of drugs are constantly being investigated. Radiation therapy at this stage is also frequently used to relieve bone pain or to treat other symptoms.

As with other treatments, your age, general health, and amount of disease and symptoms will help you decide on a specific treatment. There are also a number of clinical trials available to consider if you are facing this situation.

maybe a way to save a lot of money for the government, for insurance companies, and for ourselves—and I was also concerned about the long-term side effects of the drugs.

"Finally, in 1996 I tried Casodex on a trial basis. It dropped my PSA from 2.7 to 0.56. Understand that 2.7 was still considered normal because I still have my prostate. I finally stopped taking the Casodex, have no symptoms, and my liver functions are normal. As of July 1996, I'm off all medications. I'm just thankful I didn't have surgery or radiation. In the talks I've given about prostate cancer, one of the things I find that bothers me are the angry men who had surgery and radiation and are now living off this medicine. For some reason I was lucky! Maybe it was a miracle, maybe it was just the right drugs for me. I don't know."

"John was a perfect candidate for combination hormonal therapy," Rosalie told us. "They never should have pushed him into radiation." John, in fact, did start hormonal therapy in 1995 when his doctors noticed suspicious dark spots on his bone scans. That kicked off a roller-coaster ride of fluctuating PSA levels.

---

### Antiandrogen Withdrawal Syndrome

If your cancer becomes hormone resistant, withdrawing antiandrogen therapy is often the first line of defense. Twenty to 30 percent of patients on combined hormonal therapy (CHT) see a reduction in their PSA levels by discontinuing flutamide (Eulexin®) or bicalutamide (Casodex®). There is usually a good response for a limited time—lasting an average of three to four months. In some men, the response can last up to one to two years.

---

"My doctor started me on Lupron and my PSA dropped to 1.34 right away," remembers John. "But unfortunately, the therapy only worked for about eight to ten months before my PSA started to rise again. The next step was going on combination therapy with flutamide, and again my PSA dropped, and again, after about eight to ten months it started to rise again. So my doctors took me off the flutamide and my PSA dropped to 1.42. And I was doing really well for about six months, but suddenly it started going up again and it's now 2.81. Today, I've got cancer in my spine, my ribcage, and my arm. But we're holding off going back on flutamide. My oncologist said, 'Let's wait a little longer and see what happens. We can always put you on Casodex.' If I keep running true to form, the Casodex will probably bring the PSA down again. I'm still on the three-month Lupron shots, and I'm starting to get a little tenderness in my breasts. My nipples are a little sensitive—you women can understand that. And now I'm also in a clinical trial with PC SPES [Chinese herbs] through a company in California."

Like John, many of us use some form of Chinese herbal medicine. Charlie also takes PC SPES. "PC SPES are tiny little capsules that come in a bottle," he noted. "The problem is they do cost over $400 a month. But they have lots of great history in China. American technology has put Chinese herbal manufacturers up to speed with distribution, potency, and consistency. That's why they're so expensive."

"I still strictly follow the regimen of herbal therapies, vitamins, acupuncture, and nontraditional therapies of all kinds," said Virgil. "I practiced them before surgery and continued them after. In fact, right after the surgery, I drove into the city to my herbalist and got a

---

### *Don's Lemonade*

34 oz. distilled water
4 oz. fresh lemon juice
4 T. maple syrup
1 T. (heaping) cayenne pepper (work up to this amount)
5 gtts. (drops) hydrogen peroxide

---

fresh supply. I also got back into exercise. At first, I was just walking around the upstairs of the apartment; then I walked up and down, then started going outside—really trying to push my body to regain what I had been before and still retain my use of herbal medicines and therapies."

Don's treatment agenda also consists of herbal therapies, but as you'll recall, Don started his action plan with conventional hormonal therapy. "I went on Lupron and flutamide and within six months my PSA dropped from 2,448 to 10.6. Then it went down to 0.7, and then it went down to 0.1. Twelve months later it was down to 0.0! I was also interested in cryotherapy, so I went through all the bone scans, did the biopsy, and had an MRI, and everything came back negative. The doctors could not find any cancer. So against the advice of my doctor, I went off Lupron. My doctors said I should stay on it for the rest of my life, but I said no—kind of like Bud. I decided to be a guinea pig, too, and see what happens. So at this point, I've been off hormonal therapy for better than two years and four months. In the meantime, I had hired a biochemist-nutritionist who I continue to see once a month. Through my biochemist, I've gotten involved with ozone therapy.

"Let me tell you about my first ozone treatment," continued Don. "Man, stuff came out of my lungs like you couldn't imagine. [We can now, Don.] I spit and I frothed. My lungs must have been loaded from all my forge work as a farrier, smoking, and stuff. Anyway, this treatment really cleansed my lungs.

"But for me, the hydrogen peroxide is really an important part of all this," emphasized Don. "I started this therapy as soon as I went off the combination hormonal. I use 35 percent hydrogen peroxide in distilled water, which is part of my oxygen therapy. I mix my own water, and on the advice of my biochemist, we also started on the lemonade."

"I drink the lemonade in the morning and then switch to distilled water with 35 percent hydrogen peroxide in the afternoon. In total, I drink one-half my body weight in ounces of distilled water or lemonade a day. That's what it takes to wash the cells and make my body function properly. The theory is that cancer cannot survive oxygen—so you want to keep a lot of it in your body. And I will probably always do this. In fact, when we were all singing together last night—that's also oxygen therapy!"

(There was a grand piano at the mansion where we held our retreat, and the musicians among us gravitated to that spot in the evenings. With Charlie at the piano and Bob leading us in song, we created a few Kodak moments and musical memories. We impressed the heck out of a few of the other guests, as well!)

"I also went the magnetic bed route," Don continued. "They're made in Japan, and my biochemist recommended I try one. They had one in the office, so I laid down on that bed for an hour and a half; you can get eight hours rest on this bed in an hour. I laid on that bed, and I'm telling you, I could have driven all night. I felt so energized. So I bought one. It's magnetic, it's computer operated, and I sleep on this every night."

Magnetic bed?!! The grilling immediately began.

**Virgil:** How much does it cost?

**Don:** I bought it used. It cost me $1,000.

**Virgil:** What does it do?

**Don:** It has magnetics in it. It has little wires that go to it, and it kinda just charges the body, electrically. Your body runs on electrical impulses, and it gives you extra energy. It lets you rest. When you have a chronic problem, you gotta rest the body. It might be $1,000 down the drain, but it's worth trying.

**Paul:** I'm an electrician, and as I understand it, magnetic things are generally responsive to iron. How does a magnetic field help the cancer?

**Don:** I've been told that magnetic fields help heal bone. So do batteries.

**Paul:** We're talking about magnetics and batteries, which are two different things.

**Don:** This runs on a nine-volt system. And what you're doing is you're supposedly energizing the body. I don't get into the specifics. That's why I hired the biochemist.

**Paul:** You're going purely on a testimonial?

**Don:** No, not necessarily. If you could see what these magnetic blankets and magnetic leg wraps do for horses—how some of these horses improve. You bring them back with magnetics. I have customers who have these beds, too. Some of them are not computer operated like mine is. Some are just magnetic beds.

"And I have to say one thing regarding biochemistry and this kind of lifestyle," Don continued. "My wife and I both get tested. It costs about $40 for this kind of information, which is not much when you compare it to the cost of a doctor's visit. I get tested every month. Each test consists of a urine and saliva sample, and every month I get a computerized printout of my body chemistry. This way I can take my vitamins and minerals according to what my body needs, so I'm not just blasting it with anything and everything or megadosing on something my body doesn't need. I'm working on specific problems like my body pH and my immune system. This is preventative maintenance as far as I'm concerned. Here's what I need to do and eat. These are things I shouldn't do. For example, I ate a roll last night with dinner. And I'm still kicking myself because I feel like my digestive system doesn't work properly and it wrecks my immune system. It's also believed that cancer patients have low selenium levels. OK. If you have low selenium, doesn't it make sense to bring your selenium up to normal?

"It's really quite simple when you get into it," Don assured us. "And all the symptoms I had with hemorrhoids, the terrible prostate, the dizziness, all went away. I can't pinpoint exactly what treatment or therapy helped. It's probably the combination of hormonal therapy, detoxification, hydrogen peroxide, nutrition, everything. And I completely changed my diet. When I first started I was eating my bacon and biscuits and all this kind of stuff, and I tell you what, when I went on this program, I dropped about 20-some pounds real quickly. And I did this cold turkey. I felt bad for about two weeks. I could hardly walk a mile and had no power at all, but I kept on working. And all of a sudden my strength started coming back. And it got to be a real challenge. The more I do of this, the bet-

*Selenium.*  Selenium is a metal found in the body. It acts as an antioxidant by protecting cell membranes from attack by free radicals. It also reacts with toxic metals such as mercury, cadmium, and arsenic to form biologically inert compounds. There is also a correlation between night vision and the selenium content of the retina; the higher the selenium content, the better the vision.

ter I like it. And I have to say, again, that my wife, Lynne, supports me 100 percent and has been a tremendous help to me all along."

"I try to be helpful with his diet," responded Lynne, "and thinking up ways to make it easier for him to carry food. I started out making his lemonade and doing everything. This is a man whose cooking consisted of saltine crackers, peanut butter, and bologna. That was it. He couldn't do anything in the kitchen. Now he makes his own lemonade. He has a system worked out in the hotel rooms. He goes ahead and can find the right things to eat on his own if I'm not there."

"I don't profess to anybody that this is the way to go, but this is the way I went," concluded Don. "If I can feel this good—for me—I wouldn't ever change. It's a complete change of lifestyle. And my energy level is really great now. I get my vitality tested every month by my biochemist. My vitality potential is 100. Right now it's about 89. And it was lower, much lower, before I started all my alternative therapies. You take care of your car, your house, but your body? This is God's temple. You should take care of it."

Manuel wanted to know if Don's biochemist approved of his taking Lupron®. "He didn't really care for it too much," Don answered. "That's why if it hadn't been for the alternative methods, I would not have dared go off the Lupron. I guess I'll find out what happens. I'm still using ozone, still using hydrogen peroxide. I can go on higher doses of peroxide with no problem. I'll try variations of these things first. And I still have the option of going back on Lupron and flutamide. I'm just trying different methods. I still have all my body parts, and they're all working. And even though my PSA is starting to go up a little bit, I still have options."

"I looked at external radiation as a possible treatment option," Bob remembers, "and proton-beam radiation, which was very expensive. But as I said, I chose to have seed implants [brachytherapy].

It was a very quick procedure. They take seven needles and put them in the perineal area, and through a sonogram they guide these in. With the seven needles, they implant 70 little seeds, each smaller than a grain of rice, right into the prostate itself. There's nothing there, no swelling, no bleeding, nothing. I went into the hospital about 1:00 in the afternoon, and I was back home by 7:00 that evening, catheterized. The next morning I went back to the hospital. They took the catheter out and gave me some pills to help as far as the urination was concerned. The problems with urination went on for about two weeks, and that was demeaning—very demeaning.

"I'm a vocalist and I was performing at the time that I had my procedure done. The other fellows in the band didn't know it, but I'm standing at the microphone singing with this great big Pampers on—in my tuxedo—and I had to go to the restroom regularly to change it. I could not, in the very beginning, hold my urine, so I had to wear the Pampers. That's another thing. It's all mental. You deal with these things. I'm presenting this image of a singer up front and being Mr. Cool and whatever, and you can't tell somebody you're wearing this big Pampers. So my occupation and my performing caused some adjusting in my attitude.

"The only other side effect I had was that I was weak and I couldn't do a lot of walking. If I did a little yardwork or something I got very tired, and I had to stop. And I know that was the effect of the power of the radiation being very strong at that time. That began to wear down after several weeks, and I began to regain my energy, and I started to resume a normal life like before."

"It took me six months to regain my continence," Virgil told us. "That was probably the toughest psychological thing to deal with because my image of myself is a very strong man, and the idea of having to wear a diaper—I really suffered at that. It really had a strong impact on my image of who I was. I felt helpless. I felt disgusting and disgusted, and Manuel kept telling me over the Internet, 'Don't worry, it's going to be fine. You'll wake up one day and you'll be dry'—and ultimately I was."

"Virgil's right," Bob continued. "After I gained my energy back, which took about two weeks, there was also no incontinence. I was not impotent, and I was back just the way I was before I had the procedure done. I lost absolutely nothing, and I'm really happy with the procedure and the way it's happened. As far as sex is concerned, my doctor told me that when you climax, the ejaculation might contain

> If you choose to have brachytherapy (seed implants), your doctor will give you specific instructions about any precautions you'll need to take. See Chapter 2 for more on brachytherapy.

a small amount of blood in the very beginning, the first couple of times. After that, it clears up and everything is back to normal."

Paul added an interesting comment, "I've heard some doctors say that the seeds come out sometimes, and one of the things they do is have you urinating through a sieve, to catch any loose seeds."

"I did have a urologist check the seeds to see if they were all in place," Bob answered. "I did this about a week or two after the procedure just to make sure they hadn't slipped or come out. I also have to say that my doctor had an excellent bedside manner. He called me continually after the procedure, and this is important because we talked about educating our doctors on their bedside manner. He called me for three or four days after the procedure, and I looked up one day and he was at my door! He came to visit me and had a little bouquet of flowers! I thought, 'I don't believe this!' Wonderful guy, a young man with a great approach. You *want* to have this thing done by him. He just spoon-feeds you, stays with you right through it. It was a wonderful, wonderful procedure."

Things were not so wonderful for Peter. Peter has had his share of problems and disappointments. "My one anger really goes back to the misdiagnosis before I was treated. I didn't get any treatment for several years because of urologists who didn't diagnose what I had as being cancer. Later on I found out that my urologist never did radicals. I didn't know that. I think it was one of the reasons he failed to take it to that point, because he wasn't qualified to continue on and give me the treatment that was considered the gold standard in Sarasota at that time.

"Before I had surgery, I went out and worked like heck—got to walking five miles a day, lost ten pounds, and really put myself in pretty good shape before I gave my blood. So I went into surgery with a very positive attitude. I was first diagnosed at either Stage B or C with a Gleason score of 5, and my PSA was 17.5. So for me, surgery was a potential cure, and in May of 1990, I had a radical prostatectomy. My lymph nodes were negative and the seminal vesicles were also negative, but they were taken out as well as my prostate.

## Hormonal Therapy: How Long Will It Work?

Hormonal therapy is an effective therapy in advanced prostate cancer and may control the disease for many years. In fact, it reduces PSA levels in 99 percent of men. However, because some cancer cells are not responsive to hormonal therapy or become resistant, hormonal therapy usually stops working at some point in time. When that happens is different for every individual. The cancer cells are now called refractory to that particular type of therapy.

The cancer cells will multiply and your PSA levels will begin to rise—either within a short amount of time or sometimes not until years later. That's why it's important for you and your health care provider to keep track of your PSA regularly—so that changes can be made in therapy if needed. Some men find it helpful to keep a personal chart of their PSA levels. If hormonal therapy has stopped working for you, there are other therapies you can consider.

"After surgery, I immediately became a Stage C because the cancer had escaped the capsule. From an emotional and psychological standpoint, that was devastating. That's not what you want to hear. That's not what I'd like to know right now, but it was a fact. I am someone who can usually accept something factual—something that I can't change. I seem to be better able than some people to accept it and say OK now that's fact, now what am I going to do? Not to change it, because I can't, but what am I going to do to go on with my life in spite of this fact that I have to accept? I think that's probably helped me in this whole process.

"For two and a half years I was clean—meaning my PSA was not measurable," continued Peter. "Then it started to rise, and because I was fairly young, had a family and a business, my urologist recommended that I have external radiation, although he did tell me that the chances were only one in a thousand that it would help. I did go through radiation in 1992, with some damage, but not severe, like John. Unfortunately, it didn't help and my PSA rose quite rapidly after that. I think it was first measurable as 1.4 and within nine months it was at 6.9. So at that point, I started consulting with an oncologist. First, we tried an experimental drug called Calcitrol, which didn't work at all. Within 30 days, my PSA started rising, so we started CHT in July of 1993. I did have severe hot flashes with that. Fortunately, they're not as severe now because I take Megace. I used to take a couple 20-milligram pills a day. Now I'm down to one. So that's been one continuing aftereffect of the treatments I've had.

"So I'm just beyond three years with CHT," Peter told us, "and my PSA has not been measurable since. My current PSA level is less than 0.1, which means it's not measurable. And again, I have to say that I was very positive going into all this. I'm sorry the first therapy failed, but I was glad there was another avenue, which was radiation. But it failed, too. I knew going on CHT that the chances were 99 out of 100 that it would work. But I also knew it wouldn't work forever. So for me, surgery was a potential cure; radiation was supposedly a potential cure; CHT is not. It won't last forever. It's just something to give me some additional time. And even though the outcome of the surgery was not good, I'm glad I did it. And I'm glad I prepared myself physically, because it was the right thing to do. It not only helped me physically but, I think, mentally, too, because I felt that I was doing something to contribute to the effort we were making."

At that time, Bob said something that a lot of us were thinking. "One of the worst influences on our thinking is that doctors convince you that you should have radiation. Then it fails, but the aftereffects of the radiation are sometimes worse than the failure of the radiation."

"My side effects weren't that severe," Peter responded. "I had some aftereffects, but they were short term, mostly a lot of bowel irritation at the time. My worst segment was the last couple weeks of therapy and the following couple of months. I was in pain and I had some continuing problems, but again, not significant."

"Just remember that everyone is different," reminded John. "Even today I've got to be very careful, and I had the radiation back in 1992."

If you're faced with a decision of whether to have radiation, you'll need to talk it over with your doctor. It may, in fact, be the best option for you. It's a very personal decision, as all these treatments are.

"I went on hormonal therapy first, Lupron and flutamide, for seven months," Derek began, "and after seven months I thought I might be clear. But a biopsy showed that there was still something suspicious in my prostate. And that was confirmed about three weeks later by another lab report. Both labs said they couldn't quite make out what was there. 'Maybe it's cancer,' they said, 'we don't really know. It's kind of weird.' In retrospect, I probably should have said, 'Let's just stay on hormonal therapy for another three months and see what happens,' but I was tired of running around the country and of being impotent. So I decided to go ahead and do the cryotherapy. I thought cryo was the least problematic. It would be over in a day and I'd be back to normal. And if something happened that I could no longer perform sexually, my lady and I would just have to talk it out. I was very devastated with my social and my sexual relationship because I had thought about and wanted to be with this woman for 30 years. And then we finally find each other, get back together, and prostate cancer enters the scene. I couldn't do anything about it—it had to be handled. We started to wonder, 'Why are the heavens mad at us?' Anyway, as far as the procedure, the operation, everything went fine. You go in, they put you to sleep, you wake up. You're a little bit sore and you've got a little bag to drain the urine, but you have no pain and no long, extended stay. I was out the next day. I didn't have any problems with the cryo. My doctor used thermal detectors to make sure the freezing was going the way it was supposed to go. In fact, one of the five probes failed, and so the doctors had to refreeze that area, which is why it's so important that your doctors use the detectors to make sure that the freezing is accurate and that they're not leaving any cancer."

"I was out the same day, too," Paul said. Paul also had cryotherapy, but as you'll recall, he chose to have an orchiectomy first, which makes Paul's therapy a little unusual. "I really didn't know what my options were when I decided to go ahead and have the orchiectomy. I thought, 'Well, gee, I'm going to turn into a real nice person, soft, gentle, and kind,' but I don't think that happened."

"It came to the point where he knew it was either going to be a radical or he was going to have to have an orchiectomy," Phyllis interjected. "Those were basically the only two options he was given by the urologist. It would depend on what the lymph node testing showed as to which he would have. Since it had traveled to the nodes, he decided to have the orchiectomy. Before that, we didn't understand that there was a support group, and he hadn't found any information on the computer. We were just sort of traveling this journey blind."

"In retrospect, I look at myself as a four-year survivor," continued Paul, "and the orchiectomy probably was a good operation for me costwise. Now I don't have to go once a month to somebody or every three months and have a shot. And in the event that I'm proven cancer free down the road, I have the option of either taking minimal testosterone shots or possibly having a testicle transplant. But backtracking, I had the orchiectomy, and my PSA, which was 440 prior to my surgery, dropped to about 4 in about seven months' time. In the meantime, I had been fiddling around with my computer, and I got the word that I needed to get on flutamide. When I finally got on it, my PSA went down to less than 0.4, which in the Northwest is about as low as it's measured. It varies depending on the part of the country you're in. At any rate, I stumbled around some more on the computer and heard about cryotherapy. I decided to try and get rid of as much cancer in my body as I possibly could, and in 1993, I had cryo performed. And like Derek said, the procedure is a piece of cake. The only thing is, you have a tube coming out of your abdomen that drains your bladder, and that's removed after a week or so."

John brought up an important point. "We've had a lot of talks on cryo at our US TOO support groups because we've had some very good successes with it. But by the same token, each and every one of the doctors said that if the cancer breaks through the capsule and it's invaded the lymph nodes [stage D1], they will not do cryo. What I understand with you, Paul, is that they did the cryo even though they already knew that it had broken through the capsule."

"That's right," Paul responded. "And at the time they did mine, my gland had shrunk so badly that they could only get four probes in it because I'd been on hormonal treatment so long."

"And they still did it?" John asked.

"Yes, it was just done as a debulking procedure," said Paul. "Let me just add that with the cryo, I'm hoping to avoid any urination and bleeding problems if my cancer returns and gets progressively worse."

"One of the problems I have with cryo is that I've heard that it will, by definition, make you impotent," added Manuel. "It will freeze your nerve bundles and that's it—you're gone. In fact, I've heard that something like 80 percent of cryo patients lose their sexuality."

"Well, I still don't have full erections," Derek answered. "Neither the pump nor the injections did the job that they were supposed to do, and I'm still looking for different treatments. I don't have a complete loss, though. The nerve system is still there, but it's just not good enough."

---

### Research Update

The age-adjusted rate of radical prostatectomy, the most common treatment of early (nonmetastatic) prostate cancer, increased almost sixfold between 1984 and 1990. This increase was due in part to reported improvements in postoperative sexual potency after the use of newly developed "nerve-sparing" procedures.

However, published estimates of impotence following various types of radical prostatectomy may be inaccurately low, since not all patients may report treatment-related complications accurately and completely to their doctors. In contrast, direct surveys of patients indicate much higher rates of postoperative sexual and urinary dysfunction. The study says that one problem with most physician and patient surveys is that they have been performed retrospectively, and pretreatment impotence and incontinence prevalent in older men cannot be assessed accurately in this way.

This study was initiated in 94 men to assess treatment-related effects of impotence and incontinence. The patients completed questionnaires about sexual and urinary functions before surgery and at 3 and 12 months after surgery.

Data showed that nerve-sparing prostatectomy, particularly when performed unilaterally (on one side), improves postoperative sexual function to a lesser extent than previously reported. The study says

*(continues)*

---

"During surgery, they took one nerve bundle," recalled Peter, "so I had impotence problems following the surgery—not complete—but I was having problems. And now that I'm on Lupron, that has killed the libido. My wife and I handle that as well as we can in the face of my being impotent. It's not something we like because the sexual part of my life and our union was tremendous—so its loss is felt. But again, it's something factual, and somehow I'm able, and I think she is, too, to say, 'Well, that's too bad, but that's the way it is.' So you go on from there. The radiation damage is inconsequential at this point. I really don't feel that I'm suffering from side effects other than the sexual dysfunction. I may suffer more from the raft of medications that I take for my hypertension and diabetes."

Impotence and sexuality are subjects that we'll discuss in greater depth later in this book. However, they're topics that generated a lot

**Research Update** *(continued)*

that some of the previously reported benefits of nerve preservation may be the result of doctors selecting patients who are younger with less advanced cancer and not the technique per se. Men with large and more advanced cancers are offered the technique less often.

The study also says that despite younger age, better preoperative sexual function, and favorable prognosis, patients receiving nerve-sparing radical prostatectomy had little evidence of better preserved postoperative sexual function. And despite some improvement between 3 and 12 months after surgery, few men reported erections adequate for intercourse at 12 months regardless of surgical techniques. Researchers found no evidence of any benefit after only unilateral nerve preservation, which composed most of the nerve-sparing procedures in this study. Researchers also unexpectedly found that patients who underwent nerve-sparing more often reported greater urinary incontinence.

Given the apparently limited efficacy of nerve-sparing prostatectomy in preserving potency and the potential risk of leaving cancer cells behind, researchers believe nerve-sparing prostatectomy should be used judiciously, particularly if only the unilateral procedure is possible.

Source: J. A. Talcott, P. Rieker, K. J. Propert, J. A. Clark, K. I. Wishnow, K. R. Loughlin, J. P. Richie, P. W. Kantoff. Patient-reported impotence and incontinence after nerve-sparing radical prostatectomy. *Journal of the National Cancer Institute* 89, 15 (1997):1117–1123.

of talk and, for some of us, a lot of anger and frustration. For that reason, they warrant at least some discussion here.

"Physical, psychological, and emotional. I see all three angles coming at once," Manuel told us. "Both of my nerve bundles were spared in surgery, and I recovered from incontinence in about three months. But for all practical purposes, I am sexually impotent. I have erections that began about eight months after surgery, but they are of very poor quality and grossly inadequate. None of the alternatives presented to me before surgery, including the vacuum device or injection therapy, worked reliably in my case. I am a very angry person, and I feel cheated by life. It is an anger that eats me up for having lost my sexuality. My ex-wife and I struggled in a dysfunctional marriage that lasted 25 years. I divorced, remarried, and had a total communion with my second wife, Mary. But my sexuality is gone!! The anger is overpowering, and it is an anger that I cannot recover from."

"Manuel's in between jobs," Mary told us, "and I think that's part of the problem, too. So much energy is being focused into the anger that there's not enough emotional energy to go anywhere else."

"Our world is so sexually oriented," commented Paul. "When we watch TV, they're selling cars with sex. And I'm a very sexually driven person. So for me, I ended up with a great big void in my life, too. And I think this is where breast cancer and prostate cancer really differ, in the loss of sexuality."

"I used to believe like you, but I changed my mind," Manuel answered. "The sexual implications in breast cancer are horrendous because the woman can go through menopause. I, too, had the perception that you had. I thought women had it made. They lost a breast, right, but they didn't lose their sexuality. Wrong! They can, and the emotional impact can be just as devastating."

"For a woman—her breasts are like our penis," observed Virgil, "because in so many ways, so much of what is defined as the female stereotype is breast-oriented in our culture. So when you take away that, you take a woman's ability to lactate, to nurture children. There's a lot more attached to it. So it's like for you not being able to feel like a man—they feel less of a woman. Consequently, that screws up your mind as far as any sexual activity is concerned. Man or woman."

"Taking into consideration my age, stage, and Gleason score, I believe that a radical prostatectomy was really the only way to go for me," concluded Manuel. "Even knowing what I know today and what the consequences would be, I would do it again. In fact, just prior to choosing a treatment—whatever it was going to be—I knew I was going to lose my sexuality regardless. One way or the other, the risk was there. And eventually, it actually happened."

But as we all observed—even with all the side effects and aftershocks—we're all here, we're alive, and we have alternatives. Each of us made a choice. Were there any regrets? You bet. But for many of us, there was also satisfaction in believing that we had made the right choices. In any event, life goes on—and we are living it to the best of our ability. "Taking out the cancer opened a door of opportunity," said Virgil. This statement could have come from any one of us.

This is a letter Peter sent to his new doctor after his surgery. It expressed how he was feeling, his apprehensions, and his thirst for knowledge. It is just as relevant today and could be addressed to any doctor who treats prostate cancer patients.

*July 1, 1990*
*To: Dr. ———*
*From: Peter Stults*
*Subject: QUESTIONS, CONCERNS, and CONFUSIONS, which I would like to ask you to help me start resolving when I meet with you on July 6.*

*When I went into my June 15 meeting with Dr. ———, I was feeling really good about how well I was doing in recovering from surgery; so much so that I even asked him whether I should be describing my situation as "having had cancer" (past tense), or as "having cancer" (present tense).*

*A few minutes later I learned that there wasn't any question about whether I was a "had been" or a "was now" cancer patient. Rather, the all important question was whether I'll be among the 70% of my "type and stage and grade" who will die within the next five years, or the 30% who will have the opportunity to start working on their next five year experience with life.*

*Now that I know my life is at serious risk, with the statistical odds "against" me, my focus has changed on almost everything, including the acquisition of a major appetite for information. I know 1000 times as much about cancer as I did 60 days ago (I was about as ignorant as they come), but I feel that I need to acquire 1000 times more to maximize my chances of being in the "survivor" group.*

*I also feel the need to know much more about my specific condition. What is my type of cancer, type of cell, stage and grade, and what do they all mean? And what further treatment limitations apply to me compared to the other men in this already unattractive "70% group" because of the tumor (1) being "poorly differentiated" instead of "well defined," (2) having a Gleason score of 7, and (3) not having received radiation prior to surgery to minimize the spreading of cells during surgery, because we didn't know that the malignancy had gotten outside the capsule until the operation was in progress?*

*What do I need to know? How can I improve my chances of being in that 30% group instead of the majority? What should I be reading, thinking, eating? How do you do "imaging"? Where can I get good training in meditation, and nutrition, etc., etc.? And since I cannot do it all at once, what are the priority items; i.e., which ones can I afford to "put off" for a while?*

*What do I need to learn about various treatments so that I am able to make informed decisions? How useful is the PDQ analysis I have read about (and do you and your associates use it), and should I (or you) be suggesting the use of a Multidisciplinary Tumor Review board before we proceed further, etc., etc., etc.?*

*(Sometimes I feel like a grammar school student who's been abruptly transported into the M.I.T. School of Engineering at the Doctoral level, and is having to immediately start making critically important decisions with a seriously inadequate database; except that in this case, the "critically important" decisions are ones that may be life or death decisions for me.)*

*I know I can't ask you or anyone else to be responsible for giving me all the answers. If you could do that you'd be sitting "up there" on your throne. On the other hand, I'm not the first person who has had to face these problems while under your care, and I like what I've heard and felt from you in our few face-to-face meetings and in the "Man-to-Man" sessions I've attended, especially relative to the importance of (1) the Doctor/Patient relationship, (2) the patients' participation in treatment and (3) the mutual belief by both Doctor and Patient that the treatment decided upon is going to work.*

*I haven't met Dr. ———, and while I like and have great respect for Dr. ———, I don't see him (at least for me), as the "Bernie Siegel" type of physician I think I should have as my "Medical Manager." I'm hoping you will be willing and able to take on that role: offering suggestions and guidance (and/or an occasional well placed kick when appropriate) from the experiences you've had.*

*I would like you to be the "Bernie Siegel" member of my support and treatment team. Will you accept? I'll do my best to be one of your ". . . exceptional patients."*

*In any event, I look forward to meeting with you on Friday.*

Note: Bernie Siegel is a physician who writes inspirational books on healing.

TABLE 4.1  Book Contributors and Summary of Their Disease and Treatments

| | Date Diagnosed | Age at Diagnosis | Stage | Grade | PSA | Treatment | Complementary Therapies | Nutrition | Current Stage and PSA (1996) |
|---|---|---|---|---|---|---|---|---|---|
| Paul | 8/92 | 59 | D1 | 10 | 440 | 9/92 Orchiectomy<br>1993 Flutamine<br>1993 Cryosurgery | | No sugar for diabetes | D1<br><0.4<br>Metastasis to lymph nodes |
| Bud | 12/89 | 67 | C2, D1 | | 79 | 1/90 CHT<br>10/90 Stopped CHT<br>1991–1996:<br>Intermittent therapy<br>1996 Casodex<br>7/96 No therapy | | | 2.6 |
| John | 10/91 | 67 | B1 | 6 | 182 | 10/91 Tumor removed; prostate not removed<br>12/91 Radiation<br>1995 13 more radiation treatments<br>1995 CHT | PC SPES (Chinese herbs), Essiac tea | Low cholesterol for heart condition | D2<br>3.8<br>Hormone refractory<br>Metastasis to to spine, rib-cage, left arm |
| Charlie | 8/91 | 65 | D3 | 5 | 12 | 9/90 TUR<br>8/91 RP<br>7/93 Hyperbaric chamber<br>12/94 CHT | PC SPES (Chinese herbs), Essiac tea, citrus pectin, vitamins A, D, natural supplements (garlic, protein energy supplement), distilled water | Low fat, vegetarian, lots of fresh fruit, water, brown rice | D2<br>3.3<br>Hormone refractory<br>Metastasis to pelvic bone |

*(continues)*

TABLE 4.1  (continued)

| | Date Diagnosed | Age at Diagnosis | Stage | Grade | PSA | Treatment | Complementary Therapies | Nutrition | Current Stage and PSA (1996) |
|---|---|---|---|---|---|---|---|---|---|
| Virgil | 6/95 | 49 | B2, T2c | 6 | 7.4 | 9/95 RP | Chinese herbs, acupuncture, vitamins, other herbal supplements | Low fat, no red meat | <0.1 |
| Peter | 3/90 | 59 | B or C Post-op: C | 5 / 7 | 14.5 / 17.5 | 5/90 RP 11/92 Radiation 6/93 Calcitrol 7/93 CHT | | Low fat, low sugar for daibetes | D or D1 <0.2 |
| Manuel | 7/94 | 55 | B, T2 | 7 | 5.2 | 8/94 RP | Antioxidants (vitamins A, C, E, selenium, zinc) | Low fat, whole grain cereals, fruits, vegetables, legumes, no red meat, fish and poultry in small portions | B <0.15 |
| Bob | 8/93 | 63 | B1 | 6 | 8.5 | 8/93 Saw palmetto 2/95 Brachytherapy (seed implants) | | Low fat/no fat, fish, fruits, vegetables | 0.54 |
| Derek | 9/92 | 62 | B1-B2 | 9 | 11.8 | 8/93 CHT 3/94 Cryosurgery | | Low fat, vitamins, minerals | 0.6 |
| Don | 4/93 | 57 | D | 8 | 2,448 | 4/93 CHT (1 year) | Vitamins, distilled water with hydrogen peroxide, ozone, colonic, chiropractic, biomagnetics | Low fat, fruit, steamed or fresh vegetables, brown rice, legumes | D 3.8 |

# 5

# *Living with Prostate Cancer*

*If I had my choice I'd go back and not have this happen, but nevertheless, there is a good deal of good that has come out of my diagnosis—which both surprises and pleases me. I see it in this group here, today.*

—*Peter Stults*

When you spend practically every waking hour together for five days, you get to know one another pretty well. You talk about the good times and the bad, what makes you happy, what makes you sad. In fact, you get to know the other person's innermost feelings— and you get to understand your own. You become friends. That's what it was like for us to participate in this book retreat. But trust us—it wasn't all work (although some might argue that point); and with a unique group like ours, there's no way we would have allowed it to be.

We mentioned earlier that evenings were often spent socializing with each other and with some of the other guests staying at the mansion. Manuel summed up the essence of the retreat with this story, "Last night, a woman was singing with us during one of our sing-alongs in the living room. She asked me what we were all doing here. So I told her that all of us had prostate cancer and that we were here having a seminar to gather information for a book. She looked at me for a minute in total disbelief, and she said, 'My God, you sure know how to have a good time!' She probably thought we all had to start buying coffins."

Nothing could be further from the truth. In fact, we think you'll find that getting on with your life will become top priority. But in

*Testosterone.* This male hormone is essential for your sex drive. Many men who have undergone an orchiectomy or who are on hormonal therapy to lower testosterone levels say they don't feel quite "normal." They report feeling irritable and less aggressive. Others report weight gain, loss of muscle mass, and subtle changes in skin tone and hair growth. (P. C. Walsh, J. F. Worthington. *The Prostate.* Baltimore, MD: Johns Hopkins University Press, 1995, 156.)

the beginning, you may find that you and your disease are one and the same.

"Prostate cancer molds your life," Manuel told us. "It can become a big part of your personality. It never goes away from you. In other words, once I was given the news, it changed me."

And it will probably change *you.* Dealing with this disease and the side effects of some of the treatments can change you psychologically and physically. You may find your clothes getting a little tighter because of weight gain, especially if you're receiving hormonal therapy. Or you may find yourself losing weight if you're battling the latter stages of this disease. You and your significant other may notice mood swings and bouts of sadness, anger, and fatigue. You may experience breast tenderness or find yourself trying to adjust to the inconvenience and devastation of incontinence and/or impotence—even if these conditions are temporary. And depending on your stage and treatment, pill taking may become permanently programmed into your daily routine.

"It's important to learn to live *with* prostate cancer so you can maintain your sanity," emphasized Peter. "For example, every eight hours I take flutamide, but it doesn't remind me that I have prostate cancer. Now, it's just part of my routine. Every eight hours I take these two pills, but it doesn't really say anything to me in my brain about cancer."

Training your brain to sidestep the ever-present physical and mental cues of cancer will probably take some time. So what helps restore balance to your life after it's been twisted, tossed, and bruised up one side and down the other? "Laughing, community, business, family, relationships," we all answered at once.

"Return to whatever *you* consider to be normal," suggested Virgil. "The thing that is the key determinant in survivorship is that

> ## Research Update
>
> Studies have shown that patients with organ-confined disease have the most favorable prognosis after a radical prostatectomy. Yet up to 26 percent of patients will suffer clinical treatment failure during a 15-year follow-up period.
>
> A recent study evaluated the potential clinical and pathologic factors that predict treatment failure in patients with organ-confined and margin-negative disease. Its purpose was to define patients who may benefit from adjuvant therapy.
>
> Three hundred forty-one prostate cancer patients who had undergone a radical prostatectomy were part of the study. Patients were seen one month after surgery, then every three months for two years, and thereafter for evaluations every six months.
>
> The results of the study showed that predictors of PSA failure or treatment failure during the first postoperative year included a Gleason score of 7 or greater and a preoperative PSA level of greater than 10. Therefore, these patients should be considered for adjuvant androgen-suppression therapy (hormonal therapy).
>
> In addition, the study said that androgen-suppression therapy has a potentially curative role only if all cancer cells that remain postoperatively are androgen-dependent. It is not known if androgen independence is acquired as the disease advances or if androgen independence exists early in the natural history of the disease.
>
> Source: A. V. D'Amico, R. Whittington, S. B. Malkowicz, D. Schultz, J. E. Tomaszewski, A. Wein. Prostate-specific antigen failure despite pathologically organ-confined and margin-negative prostate cancer: The basis for an adjuvant therapy trial. *Journal of Clinical Oncology* 15 (1997):1465–1469.

you have walked away from the plane crash. Now you're going to go back and do whatever it is that you've been doing before or whatever else different you choose to do. You've dealt with the crisis, you've dealt with the beast, and you've beaten it back. You've got a rapport with it that's going to allow you to go forward and do what *you* want to do. I'm always aware that I've got it, that it's there. But I don't wake up every morning thinking, 'How am I going to fight prostate cancer today?' What I've done is make changes in my life that say, if I do this, I should become healthier. I should become more well. There are things I've done advocacy-wise that have helped my mental state to help promote my battle, but I don't take it out of bed with me, hold it by its hand, and say, 'Let's go out together.' I do dismiss it to a great extent."

Not treating the disease as a constant companion is perhaps easier to do if you were diagnosed at an earlier stage. For those of us who have faced treatment failures, prostate cancer is perhaps a little more difficult to dismiss. There is no cure for metastatic/hormone-refractory prostate cancer. We are always aware of that. As Charlie told us, "I'm constantly looking for new treatments and constantly changing treatments to try and stay ahead of this disease."

"I had to make a conscious effort," said Peter. "I can't tell you exactly how I did it, but I'm aware that I sort of worked to get it out of being all-consuming—so that I wasn't thinking about it every night when I went to bed and I wasn't thinking about it every morning. I guess I probably did this through substitution—finding other things, finding my 'normalcy,' and focusing on those things that are important in my life such as family and community, and pushing prostate cancer in the background, where I think it's important for it to be most of the time."

"In my case," explained Virgil, "I was forced to not have it be an issue by the nature of my work. Getting back into my business life, it seemed like people really didn't care that I had prostate cancer. 'Oh, yeah,' they'd say. 'How do you feel, Virg? Good?' They really don't care. So it's very easy not to think about it because nobody else is thinking about it. Nobody else is going to be sympathetic, so you've got to just get back into the swing of it. Do what you have to do."

"I just pretty much tried to focus on my work, too," said Don, "and when I was busy shoeing horses, I wouldn't think about prostate cancer. But people were concerned about me. Sometimes I'd be between horses, and somebody would come into the barn and want to talk about it or ask how I was doing."

"I think Don's in a different type of situation from Virgil," Lynne smiled. "That's because people who have horses are nicer people. The people Don deals with probably have more empathy and caring and interest in other people than the business world does!"

"My situation was a little different, too," said Peter. "I was president and owner of my own company. So after my wife and I had adjusted to the diagnosis, we made an initial decision to bring in someone to replace me. I called my employees together and announced it and, yes, that was difficult. It was an emotional thing to do, but I felt the need to let them know as opposed to trying to hide it. That was just a decision I made. And they were and continue to be interested and supportive even though I'm retired and not in the office every day. Those who've been around awhile are always curious about what my three-month checkups are like and what my PSA is."

We all agreed that life would never be the same. In fact, prostate cancer is a challenge you'll face for the rest of your life. But regardless of your stage, it is a challenge that you *can* live with and deal with.

In other words, you *never* lose sight of your cancer and the need to stay informed and empowered, but you also recognize that when it comes to this disease, tunnel vision probably won't benefit you or your family. Maybe that means taking a few steps back from the day-to-day frustrations and adjusting your focus on life.

As Charlie said—even with all the frustrations and problems he's had to deal with—"There's no ill wind that doesn't blow some good. Psychologically, I got stronger," he told us. "What cancer did was refocus my mind totally. It refocused my relationship with my children, with my family, with my clients, and with God."

"In many ways I'm a happier person now than I was before," Peter told us. "I've faced this crisis, and I've changed my value system, but not so much consciously. It's not as though I said I'm going to do this, and this, and this. I don't think I did it that way. I think that through the process of the crisis, my value system changed. Material things are not as important; relationships are much more important to me. I had tremendous support from my employees, my friends, my neighbors, my family—just a wonderful outpouring of love in all sorts of ways—which has enabled me to respond in kind, to a greater extent than I had before. So there are a lot of things about my life that are superior to what it was before."

"Once I really understood what prostate cancer was all about," Charlie said, "I also began to examine my own life—not only examine it but take charge of it. Have I changed my whole life 180 degrees? No, but I changed it 90 degrees and parts of it I did change 180 degrees. I took charge of my own life in relation to my family— my five children and my wife. My relations with my family improved because I realized that my future was uncertain for the first time. Suddenly, there was an element in my life, a disease, that was incurable and that did not exist before. So now there was a possible time lock on how long I would be around, and the important things in my life began to really pop up: my children, who have been terrific and very supportive throughout all this, and my wife. She became much more important to me. I hug her more, take her out to dinner more; the whole relationship, which has always been good, has really been enhanced. I hate to say that the disease caused that—but it did."

"Cancer is probably the best thing that's ever happened to Don," said Lynne, "and our life, our communication, and our marriage because he's much more open and he's much more willing to share feelings. He understands much more about feelings and emotions and the importance of communication than he ever did before—than he ever allowed before."

"Was he a John Wayne?" asked John.

"Absolutely," said Lynne, "Horse and all!"

"You have to realize," said Don, "that in my travels in the horse-shoeing business, I talk to a lot of people. Some of the guys are real macho, too, you know. And somebody like me, being a blacksmith, you kind of have this macho image, too. You can talk to some of these guys—others you can't. You have to feel them out when you talk to them. You have to know what to say and how much they can take."

"Emotions are very real," said Virgil. "We men oftentimes don't want to deal with that reality of ourselves. We say that's a feminine thing, and we just don't want to be emotional."

"Exactly," said Bob. "We try to maintain this image of being macho. 'It's OK. It doesn't hurt, I can handle it.' In the process of trying to keep that image up, you keep whatever little ills you have to yourself because you're looked upon as a 'wuss.' Quit whining. Just deal with it. Don't even talk about it; deal with it!"

"But in order to deal with it, you have to talk about it," answered Mary.

"That's exactly my point," continued Bob. "For example, there was a guy who worked with us on the police force. Big guy, lifted weights—there were never enough weights in the gym when he was there. He was a very, very macho guy. Well, he was diagnosed with cancer. He took some time off work, but when he came back, he had to wear a colostomy bag. While he was in uniform, he was wearing this bag around. First of all, this did a lot of things to him mentally. He couldn't cope with it, so he left work again for a couple of weeks. He came back to work without the bag. So everybody asked, 'How ya doing?' He said, 'I'm doing fine. No problem.' But he still had cancer. We had a gym on top of the station where everybody worked out and a track. One day I saw him as I was going into the lunchroom, and I spoke to him. He was sitting there just staring into space in uniform. I got my lunch, walked back out, and the next thing I know I heard this big blast. And we all ran up upstairs. He'd blown his brains out right there all over the track. But here was a guy who tried to keep working out. He tried to do everything, but he couldn't cope with it mentally. A lot of men don't talk about it—or can't talk about it. I realize now that that is wrong."

Rosalie jumped into the conversation with some perspective. "Women are trained to communicate differently than men are. Men are brought up to be competitive from the time they're little boys. This macho John Wayne thing starts to take over. Women have by nature been a support group for each other. In the colonial periods, women had their sewing circles and quilting bees, where they poured out all their frustration and disappointments, and their marital problems and child-rearing problems. We call it interfacing now. But the point is women were doing this very naturally then. Even today, whenever women have health problems, they usually feel free to talk to one another about them. John and I were appalled to find out that some of the men who come to the US TOO International meetings haven't even told their families that they have prostate cancer. The bottom line is, if you can't communicate on other levels and you're hit with a catastrophic situation where you find out that you have any kind of cancer—prostate cancer, breast cancer, lung cancer—it just exacerbates the void between the man and the woman."

One thing we all agreed on is that we are not living with cancer alone. This disease has also struck our families, and the impact on our wives and partners has probably been equal to what it has been on us.

"Sometimes, I think, wives see us as the rock that they can depend on," Virgil said. "And all of a sudden, if that rock is cracked, they can perceive that their own lives are at risk. 'What's going to happen if I don't have this guy who will be there for me?' All of a sudden, their sense of security and maybe even their sense of identity become at risk. I think we need to talk about the need to have our partner supporting us, but concurrently, we've got to be able to support them."

"I subscribe totally to what you just said," Peter added. "I was devastated by the diagnosis, but it was worse for my wife—and we've had some problems. She sort of rejected my diagnosis and went into a little cocoon. This was about six years ago, and it's gotten better, but she still has difficulty talking about it and even thinking about it.

"And I know it was really a threat to her security—and not just her security, but there was the fear of losing someone she loved and the father of her child. As I've learned more, I've become more comfortable with living with this disease even though the prognosis is not good in a classical sense. But my wife hasn't really participated a lot in learning with me. I think that's one reason that she continues to be more uncomfortable about it than I am. She's supportive but still uncomfortable with my diagnosis."

"For me," Charlie told us, "prostate cancer became an opportunity to improve relationships and to take another really good look at *myself*, a very severe look at myself and say, 'What kind of person are you and what kind of person do you want to be, what kind of reality do you want to create?' So emotionally, I got much closer to my whole family—in a very loving, caring way—and we have always been a very close, hugging family. Our children get hugged every day that we see them. You don't get out of the house without that."

"The problem is, we men were brought up *not* to hug," Bob interjected. "I started my son off that way. I'd kiss my daughters, and I'd shake his hand. I found out that was a mistake. I should have hugged my son. I should have kissed him, also. We both realize that now. We both came to the realization that this is important to do. He felt like he lost something because my daughters were getting this hugging and kissing, and he didn't get any of it. He got a handshake. After I realized that, I tried to kiss him, and he said, 'NO, dad—men don't kiss!' I taught him that, and I had to unlearn that."

"We have family hugs every time we're together," said Bud. "I really think all this helps; I really do. I'm six years living with prostate cancer now, and I'm still going. I don't know what it was. Maybe it was a miracle, maybe it was I just had the right drugs; I don't know what it was. But I'll tell you something; there are a couple of things they've never been able to separate out in business or medicine or anything else, and that's desire. We've mentioned perseverance—the other one is desire. I want to tell you. I have a great desire to live."

---

**Benefits of Exercise**

Low-intensity activities such as walking can do a lot for your quality of life. Exercise has been proven to reduce some of the nausea and fatigue that may be a result of your treatment and to boost your energy levels. Exercise can also increase your endorphin levels, and increased endorphin levels help with pain management. In addition, exercise can help you sleep better, increase your appetite, and generally make you feel better.

---

We all do. In fact, when we were diagnosed with cancer, it suddenly made us want to do everything we could to promote life—as long and healthy a life as possible. Most of us seized the opportunity to make up for some bad habits we had before the diagnoses. We found ourselves embarking on regular exercise routines and taking a very critical look at our eating habits and lifestyles.

"What I did, " Charlie explained, "was tell myself that I can react to it any way I want and that I have choices. My choice was to get stronger, exercise more, alter my diet radically. I was going to review my personality traits and alter them; I was basically going to change my lifestyle and my life plan.

"Today, I'm almost on a vegetarian diet, which helps me fight fatigue, and I exercise—two things I probably wouldn't have done before I was diagnosed. I eat a lot of fruit. I do some of my own cooking and I prepare healthy things. I don't drink liquor. I don't smoke. I don't do any of those things. If I didn't have this disease I would be one of the healthiest people you could imagine."

Charlie's viewpoint was shared by many of us.

"I feel good, I'm alert, and I'm able to do just about everything that I did before," said John. "Having had a heart attack, I was already on an exercise program, and I'm still on an exercise program. I was on a low-cholesterol diet. I'm still on a low-cholesterol diet. So when the cancer came along, it was just another thing to overcome. I just do everything I can to stay as healthy as I can. Sure I can't do everything I'd like to—I'm 72 years old, after all—but I do jog about three miles a day. I'm on my treadmill for an hour. I incline it and I work up a sweat. I'm also a napper. If I get a little tired in the afternoon, I meditate and POW! I can get a ten-minute nap and feel as if I've slept for hours."

*Fatigue.*   Fatigue is a common problem for most prostate cancer patients. It can be caused by the disease or its treatments or by a combination of the many changes your body is experiencing. Fatigue can cause an overwhelming feeling of being unable to function at work or at home—and can disrupt your life and your family's lives. Recognizing the problem and creating a balance between the energy you use and save is important. The first step is having reasonable expectations for yourself about what you can and cannot do. Your health care providers can also help you develop a personal plan to manage it.

Prevention and management:

- Take frequent, short rest periods rather than long naps. Shorter rest periods can be more refreshing and restorative.
- Don't lie in bed or sit more than you have to.
- Try to remain physically active through exercise, such as walking, which can help restore some energy, too.
- Keep a regular sleep schedule. Go to bed at the same time every night.
- Keep a regular activity schedule.
- If you are so ill that you can't get out of bed, have a family member help you with bed exercises. Ask your doctor or physical therapist about specific exercises.
- Drink plenty of fluids. This helps your balance and helps your muscles feel stronger.

"One problem I do have is that I get swelling in my legs," John continued. "When I had surgery, I had lymph nodes removed. I've had phlebitis, and I'm also on blood thinners. So I try to sit down a lot, especially at home, and to raise my legs. Then the swelling seems to subside."

"I still follow the same regimen of my own making that I did before the surgery," said Virgil, "and that consists of Chinese herbal therapies, vitamin supplements, acupuncture, and other nontraditional things. I take part of my supplements and therapies in the morning at breakfast, the other half at night when I eat." (See Table 5.1.)

In fact, most of us are keenly aware of our diets and lifestyle and also follow some pretty strict regimens. Fruits and vegetables, lots of water, and low-fat dishes were popular at the retreat. Don requested that distilled water be available to him daily.

*Lymphedema.* Lymphedema is a swelling of the extremities (legs or arms) that is caused by poor drainage of lymph fluid. Blockage can be caused by a tumor, by infection, the surgical removal of lymph nodes, or radiation to the lymphatic channels. In prostate cancer, the legs are the most commonly affected sites because it is the groin area where nodes have been removed or that has been radiated. There are degrees of swelling ranging from mild to severe. If caught early, lymphedema can be treated very effectively. Tell your health care provider immediately if you are having any swelling or discomfort such as

- a feeling of heaviness, fullness, or tightness of a leg or arm;
- rings or shoes that don't fit;
- decreased strength;
- redness or signs of infection.

Some treatments for mild-to-moderate lymphedema include elevating the swollen limb, using compression garments, and massage or physical therapy. Electric pressure pumps are sometimes used in moderate-to-severe cases.

Lymphatic drainage can also be improved by exercise. Therefore, exercise can be important in the prevention of lymphedema and its treatment. If your pelvic lymph nodes have been affected by prostate cancer or its treatment, ask your health care professional about specific leg and foot exercises. Some common recommended exercises include walking, swimming, light aerobics, low-risk bike riding, and yoga. Before starting any exercise program, you'll want to consult a trained physical therapy professional who can tailor a safe program to fit your personal needs.

"I've probably lost about 20 pounds since I changed my lifestyle," Don said. "And I've been able to maintain my new body weight real easily with the program I'm on, too."

"Don eats almost nothing but fruit until about 4:30 or 5:00 P.M.," Lynne told us. "Then he has steamed vegetables, rice and beans for dinner. I have many wonderful recipes that we use and he really does eat a variety of foods. As far as meat goes, he's only supposed to have Amish-grown chicken, fish that are not bottom cleaners, and venison, and he should only have those three times a week. We usually try and be done eating by about 6:00 P.M."

TABLE 5.1   Virgil's Complementary Therapy Daily Regimen

(Check with your doctor before starting any complementary therapies to make sure they do not interfere with any of your traditional treatments. All therapies need to be tailored to your individual needs and requirements.)

| Type | Dosage | Frequency/Comments |
|---|---|---|
| Vitamin C | 500mg | 1 capsule 3x/day, after eating; reduce amount if diarrhea occurs |
| Vitamin E | 400 i.u. | 1 capsule 2x/day |
| Vitamin B1, 2, 6, 12 | 200mg | 1 capsule 2x/day, after eating; may cause urine to be yellower |
| Selenium | 200mg | 1 capsule 1x/day |
| Saw palmetto extract (Serenoa repens) | 160mg | 1 capsule 2x/day; with food (use only in presence of enlarged prostate) |
| Calcium/magnesium | 500mg calcium 250mg magne- sium | 1x/day; should have minimum ratio of 2:1 calcium: magnesium after eating; before bedtime |
| Zinc citrate | 330mg | 1 capsule 1x/day; after eating |
| Pumpkin seed oil | 1000mg | 1 capsule 1x/day |
| Pycnogenol | 50mg | 1 capsule 2x/day |
| Chromium picolinate | 200mcg | 1 capsule 1x/day; with food |
| Echinacea | 400mg | 2 capsules 2x/day |
| Yohimbine | 1500mg | 1 capsule 1x/day; after eating; at night |
| CoQ-10 | 10mg | 1 capsule 1x/day |
| Valerian root | 450mg | When needed to relax/sleep |
| Dong Quai | 500mg | 1 capsule 1x/day |
| Soy protein (Genistein/ Diadzen/Glycetein) | 70mg | 2 tablets 2x/day |
| Aloe vera juice | 1–2oz | 1 or 2x/day mixed juice or tea |
| Water | 8oz. glass | At least 8x/day |
| UltraClear® | as directed | 4x/month to cleanse system |

"I feel great," added Don. "And I haven't missed a day's work. We heat our house with wood, and I cut all the wood myself. I'm very active. In fact, I'm stronger now than I was for years."

However, we all slid off our diets a little during those five days at the retreat. In fact, we were fed and watered quite well—morning,

*Lynne's Recipes*

### Super Veggie Supper

2 T. corn oil
1/2 tsp. dried oregano
1 clove garlic, minced
1 T. tamari sauce
1 small onion, chopped
2 c. chopped tomatoes
1 medium green pepper, chopped
2 c. kidney beans, cooked
1 1/2 c. zucchini, sliced
2 1/2 c. cooked brown rice
1/8 tsp. cayenne pepper
1/2 c. grated cheddar cheese

In large skillet, sauté onion and garlic in oil. Add green pepper, zucchini, oregano, and cayenne pepper. Cook until vegetables are tender, about 5 minutes. Add tamari sauce, tomatoes, and beans. Cover and cook on low for 3 to 5 minutes. Serve vegetables over brown rice and top with cheese. Serves 4.

### "Cream" of Cauliflower Soup

1 1/2 qts. distilled water
Dash cayenne pepper
1/2 head cauliflower, washed and chopped
2 garlic cloves, minced
2 stalks celery, washed and diced
1/4 tsp. garlic powder
1/2 onion, diced
1/4 tsp. onion powder
1/4 c. oat bran
1/2 block raw cheese, grated
1 T. tamari (optional)
3 small red potatoes, diced
1/2 tsp. basil

Boil all ingredients except cheese for approximately 2 hours or less. Turn off heat and blend with handheld electric mixer if you like a smooth, creamy texture. Mix in cheese and serve.

*(continues)*

*(continued)*

### Mexican Vegetable Burrito

1/4 c. chopped onion
1/2 c. chopped tomato
1 c. broccoli
1/4 tsp. oregano
2 T. grated carrot
Dash cayenne pepper
2 T. homemade mayonnaise
1 clove garlic, pressed
1/4 c. grated cabbage
Package corn tortillas, no additives
1/4 c. diced celery
Fresh parsley
1/2 avocado, sliced
Plain yogurt
1/2 c. alfalfa sprouts
1 green chili pepper, diced

Steam broccoli, chili pepper, and onion for 3 minutes in steamer
basket on top of stove. Add steamed ingredients to all of the above
except the mayonnaise. Spread generous amount of mayonnaise
onto the corn tortilla and fill with approximately 1/2 cup of filling.
Roll up and serve with chopped parsley and some chopped tomato
on the side. Top with plain yogurt.

noon, night, and in between. As Phyllis observed, "Paul has
changed his lifestyle drastically and is probably healthier now than
he was before the diagnosis. He stopped smoking, and he tries to eat
right, like cutting down on red meat. But here it's tough—with fine
wine and filet mignon on the menu."

Our coping skills encompass more than changes in diet and exercise, however. It's also a matter of, once again, refocusing on life and
making time for the things that make us happy. "I plan to put up a
fight against cancer," Paul began. "It isn't going to take me easily. On
the flip side, it's given me an opportunity to rethink my priorities. At
first, like many of us here, I thought, 'I'm going to die,' and so I
thought, well, maybe I should do some of those things I'd been holding off on. Since my diagnosis, I've gone to Europe three years in a

## Nutrition

For many men with prostate cancer, nutrition takes center stage as something they can do to help their bodies fight disease. In fact, good nutrition is at least as important as keeping active. It means eating a high-fiber, low-fat diet, with at least five servings of fruits and vegetables each day, and drinking plenty of fluids.

Research now points to a strong connection between diet and the incidence of cancer. The rate of prostate cancer, for example, is greatest in countries that have diets high in animal fat. Therefore, limiting or eliminating red meat from your diet may be an option for you to consider. Proper foods can also help you avoid problems with constipation, diarrhea, and incontinence.

row, which was really an accomplishment for me. And I've really enjoyed those types of things, which I'm sure would not have occurred unless I'd been diagnosed. I'd be procrastinating some more."

Paul wasn't the only procrastinator among us. "I'd been procrastinating about playing the guitar," Bob said, "and I kept saying to myself, 'Well, I'll get to that later on.' Since I got prostate cancer, I realized that later on is *now*. So I started working at it, and I'm going to work at it diligently and, God willing, I'm going to play the doggone thing before I leave this life. It gave me a sense of urgency to accomplish that. I've dedicated my time left here to doing that. I haven't mentioned the fact that I'm also an artist. I teach art to students, small children, and retired adults, and there are a lot of paintings I want to do. I was going to paint my family, and I'm gradually getting around to doing that. Now I've got grandkids, so the family's getting bigger. I figure I better start painting, and so I'm doing that, too."

"I'm having a hell of a good time, too," Derek told us. "I'm single with a special lady in my life. As I've said before, everything happened at once. I found Ramona and got prostate cancer. So we're making up for lost time. Ramona and I travel for months at a time and do all kinds of things that we want to do. One thing I'd like to do is get back to Europe, where we met in the Mediterranean, and the Middle East at some point, but other than that we've got no big plans for the future. We're just enjoying the present and having a great time together."

"Since the diagnosis," Peter said, "my wife and I have gone from two-week vacations to six-week vacations."

"We went from *no* vacations to—vacations!" Lynne told us. "Quite a few of them, in fact."

"My wife is a survivor of melanoma," Don reminded us, "so we've been through this before."

Didn't *that* precipitate lots of vacations, we all wanted to know?

"No. I guess I didn't think it was a problem or an issue," answered Don. "I figured I had to keep raking in the money to support the family. We had just built a new house, and I wanted the kids to enjoy all that. I felt that I was the breadwinner and I had to keep going because I got paid for what I do—no more. I have people who depend on me to shoe their horses from one time to the next. I'm usually booked several months in advance, and I've always felt obligated. But I guess I wasn't quite as obligated to my family as I was to my job. That was probably a mistake. So really, cancer has been a good experience in a lot of ways. I hate to say that, but it has really opened my eyes."

"You have to take time to smell the flowers," said Rosalie, "only we need to start earlier than finding we've got a life-threatening situation. Our priorities are skewed in this country."

But even if you make lifestyle changes, try to eat right and stay fit. As Paul reminded us, "We live in the real world. You go outside and all the automobile fumes go up in the air and you suck those in. You go to the store, you buy contaminated food. There are sulfites in the wine; sodium nitrites in bacon, ham, lunch meats. You drink contaminated water. Even the ozone that protects us is gone, and so we live in a contaminated world. So what do we do? Live in a glass bubble?"

"I think Paul just made a really brilliant point," said Charlie. "The environment we live in here in the United States is often poisonous. The air, the pollution, the chemicals, the food that we eat, the hormones in the food, the way meat and chicken are raised and processed, the pesticides; and Paul used the analogy of a bubble that would literally handshackle and imprison us. But I don't feel imprisoned. I feel that we, individually, reject the bubble notion."

"But there are so many things out there that you don't know about," said Bob, "that are harmful and that we use every day. You think you're doing the right thing. I take all my medications. I do all the things right, but then I eat out of this plate that's just loaded with lead. I'm using this deodorant with aluminum. I've heard that's bad for you. And I'm thinking, 'What can you do?'"

"You have to read the labels," said Don. And Lynne added, "If you can't understand the label, it's probably not good for you."

"But it's not necessarily reading labels," answered Bob. "If you pick up a plate to eat with and you find out that plate has lead in it, well, there's no label to tell you that. What about the deodorants? We're just buying whatever there is, and there's nothing on the label that tells you this is harmful."

And what about occupational hazards?

"I spent 22 years at a radar school," said Derek, "so who knows what effect that had on me?"

"I worked in a computer room for 25 years," said Manuel, "and there's been a tremendous incidence of cancer in all of us who worked in that room. We had three cases of testicular cancer that were very rare."

"And don't forget high overhead electrical tension wires," said Virgil.

"Right," said Bud. "In Michigan, there have been several lawsuits against the power companies, where the overhead electrical lines have affected the production of milk in dairy herds. The other thing I wanted to add is that if you're worried about the aluminum in deodorants, you can buy a stick-type of deodorant called Crystal Oasis that contains no aluminum. It's made from natural mineral salts and is free of any perfume or chemicals. It's available in most stores and it works great!"

Cosmic rays, microwave ovens, chlorinated water. . . . We could have gone on and on.

"There is something we *can* do about all this," Mary told us. "We *can* lobby the government to make changes as far as industrial pollution, automobile pollution, and what is put into our food supply, like the hormones that are put into the meat supply. We have these epidemic proportions of hormone-related cancers in people. But the point is, we're not totally helpless here. If you think about your disease, and you see something that you know is going to be harmful to you—you *can* do something about it."

"That's the point," said Charlie. "We have to learn to fight against that. And we may well have given ourselves cancer by our diet, stress, and behavior. I don't know. But there are ways we can minimize the rise and, hopefully, the progression, or try and avoid it. We can take charge of our lives. We can recognize that there are alternative remedies—like the terrific things that Don does. There are vitamins, exercises, and things that are considered on the 'fringe.' We need to get this message out to people, to have and trust their own judgment—but it must be informed judgment. If you have knowledge and confidence, then you'll have hope and be prepared to live in a world where there is a terrible disease and not be afraid of it. That way you'll avoid the bubble effect."

"I think the greatest continent in the world is between our ears," said Bud, "and I look at it as a garden. I think a lot about what caused this cancer. Because you can have the most beautiful garden in the world, but if you go away and leave it for two weeks, it's full of weeds when you come back. We didn't grow the weeds, but they may get in our brains, and you have to pull them out every day. You have to pull those bad thoughts out. I look back and think, gee, I was living pretty well, I was on the road giving talks on positive thinking, I was having steaks that maybe I shouldn't have had, one or two cocktails a week with those dinners, and I start thinking maybe I brought a lot of this on myself. I don't know. We just have to look inside once in a while."

Charlie had a final surprising comment on the "side effects" of staying fit, looking good, and living healthily. "The problem with my family dealing with this disease, or with anybody, is that I do look good. People say, 'God, you look great, Charlie! Haven't seen you look this good in years!' So when you don't look sick, it's hard for people to think of you as having this disease, so they can never really be on your support team."

In fact, many cancer patients find that they need to build a whole new support system of friends because some people just can't cope with the fact that you have cancer.

"People are afraid," everyone said practically at once.

"And it's not just fear that makes them uncomfortable," explained Lynne. "They don't know what to say, and so they'd rather not have to confront it and they stay away. And if there are people who are making you uncomfortable and giving bad counsel, you don't have to listen to them, and you don't have to allow them to dominate your time or your life. Go to the people who you feel are helpful. People who aren't helpful can make things worse."

"I think you're right," responded Paul. "I had some friends that I went to grade school and kindergarten with. And whether they

---

### The PSA (prostate-specific antigen) Test

As mentioned in Chapter 1, the test for PSA is not perfect but is the most sensitive marker of prostate cancer currently available and is used to help screen for prostate cancer and to monitor the effectiveness of treatments. PSA levels that are decreasing, remaining the same, or increasing all have different meanings and may suggest whether the treatment is working or should be changed. Remember, PSA is prostate specific—not cancer specific. You can have a high PSA and not have cancer or have a low PSA level and still have prostate cancer. And your PSA level can remain low while your cancer continues to grow and spread.

---

could handle it or not, I don't know, but they don't like me anymore. They've shunned me."

"They *will* shun you," said Don. "I've felt the same thing. There are people who can't look you in the eye. They look the other way. Now they see me around the basketball tournaments, and other places, still carrying on my normal activities, so that's changed some of their perceptions."

"But people ask me a lot, 'Is Don still all right?'" said Lynne. "'How's Don feeling?' They act like he's probably going to die— soon!"

"That's why it's so important to get involved, and stay involved, with support groups," said Rosalie. "People can form a whole new bonding chain through support groups, and sometimes they're better off to form new friends who will help them than to stick with old friends who are going to destroy them."

"You've got to find people who know what this disease is all about," added Charlie. "That's imperative for support people. Maybe I think about all these things more than the rest of you because my cancer is more advanced. I don't know. All I know is that it's never far from my mind."

"I don't think I ever get it out of my mind," responded Derek. "I live a perfectly great life, travel, have a good time, but I know that three months down the road I've got to have another PSA and that number keeps moving. It isn't critical yet; nor am I worried about it, but it's always in the back of my mind. What if I go in tomorrow

## Research Update

One of the major challenges in the management of prostate cancer is to correctly identify those individuals who are likely to benefit from a therapeutic intervention. A recent study identified two early prostate cancer populations within stages T1–T2ab, Gleason scores of 2 to 7, and PSAs of 4 to 15ng/ml. One hundred forty-six patients within these ranges were treated with external-beam radiation alone from November 1987 to October 1993.

The goal of the study was to identify a favorable subgroup of men for whom radiation alone is adequate therapy and an unfavorable subgroup whose outcome may justify more aggressive treatment. Data showed that although stage and Gleason score remain important predictors of relapse-free survival, pretreatment PSA levels appear to be statistically more important predictors.

Patients whose pretreatment PSAs were less than 8ng/ml had superior results with conventional radiation therapy. Ninety-eight percent of these patients reached a PSA below 1 within three years compared to only 78 percent of patients with a PSA greater than 8. In addition, with an average follow-up of 38 months, a low pretreatment PSA (4 to 8ng/ml) was directly correlated with improved relapse-free survival when compared to patients with an 8 to 15ng/ml level. These patients had a 27 percent failure rate at five years and may benefit from more aggressive treatment techniques with hormonal therapy.

Source: J. P. Lattanzi, A. L. Hanlon, G. E. Hanks. Early stage prostate cancer treated with radiation therapy: Stratifying an intermediate risk group. *International Journal of Radiation Oncology, Biology, Physics* 38, 3 (1997):569–573.

and it's up a point and a half? I'm working on it, but I certainly don't feel I'm over this."

"We're PSA addicts. We live by our PSA." Bob said it. We all understood it.

"For me, once I have the blood drawn, I start getting nervous until I know what the results are," Paul told us, "and I spend two to three days praying. Then I find out I got a good report and I'm happy as hell. Until next time."

"I'm less nervous now than I used to be," said Peter, "even though every three months that go by get me closer to the time I'm likely to have a measurable PSA. Maybe it's just because I'm accustomed to

Many men find it useful to chart their own PSA levels so they can keep their personal records up to date. Remember, however, that the PSA test is not perfect. If you chart your PSA, there are also many variables to keep in mind, including your age and the velocity, or rate of change. It's hoped that PSA velocity will become valuable in helping doctors distinguish between prostate cancer and benign prostatic hyperplasia (BPH).

the test and I know there's no point in worrying about it. I still, however, feel some anxiety each time, but much less so now. I do remember worrying a lot after my surgery and radiation both failed and I went on the CHT. For me, there was no widely accepted 'next step' after CHT—and that caused me to have some considerable concern."

Going in for your routine PSA test can be psychologically and emotionally trying, to say the least. Will it be the same number as before? Will it have gone up a tenth of a point, one point, or ten points? And should you be concerned? When *should* you be concerned? It's a numbers game that'll drive you nuts—if you let it.

"Do I think about it? You bet," said John. "Next week I have to go for a PSA, so I'm thinking, is it going to go up another four-tenths or not? There's nothing we can do about that. The big frustration is—there's no cure."

Manuel had a novel approach to dealing with THE TEST. "If I know I can get my results on a Thursday or Friday, I don't bother getting them. I call on Monday, Tuesday, or Wednesday. I don't want to possibly ruin my weekend. It's already ruined because you worry, regardless. Then you call in and they give you the good news—below 0.5—aaaahhhh! I feel like all my PSA needs to do is rise just a hair and I'm cooked. You are ruled by your PSA!" (At the time of the retreat, 0.5 meant unmeasurable. Since that time, assays have gone from 0.5 to 0.2 to 0.1. Currently there are assays used that go all the way to 0.00.)

Charlie gets his PSA checked monthly but says, "It does *not* rule my life. I agree that you live by your PSA to a certain extent, but if you're metastatic and refractory, as I am, it's a whole different drill. That's because, as John said, there's no cure. And while I have regular PSA tests, what I'm ruled by—and live by—is the progression

What matters when dealing with PSA velocity is a significant change over time. If you have an average steady increase of more than 0.75 nanograms per milliliter a year, that could signify that you have prostate cancer or that it is growing. Researchers say it could eventually help doctors make a more accurate diagnosis of prostate cancer at an earlier stage. Two points to keep in mind: At present, it's unclear what rate of change is significant in men with PSAs greater than 10, and 25 percent of men with prostate cancers that are growing do not have a big increase in their PSA. (P. C. Walsh, J. F. Worthington. *The Prostate.* Baltimore, MD: Johns Hopkins University Press, 1995.)

and spread of my disease. My PSA can be low, but my disease is still growing, and that's what I really have to be aware of."

"My PSA started rising soon after my cryotherapy," Derek told us. "So I watch it every time, and I'm always anticipating. But there's also the acceleration, or rate of rise, that you should look for. Mine's been rising, and it's only at 0.6 now, so it's not any big deal, but you still get that 'where is it?' feeling. And where's it going to be next time? It just worries me every time I have my PSA taken."

"I had an experience," said Paul, "where my PSA was 0.1, 0.1, 0.1. Then I went to a different lab to have my blood drawn, and the results came back 0.5, so I ran down to my funeral director. Not quite, but I felt like it. In reality, I was just ignorant of the importance of keeping the same lab and in learning what 'less than' really meant. Once that got through to me, why I felt a lot better."

"Worldwide, there are 64 different assays that are used for PSA," added Peter, "so unless the lab comes back and states which assay they used, it really is meaningless, and confusing for doctors. You get different results from different labs."

"There was also a completely different PSA test being done back in 1990," Bud told us. "One of the current assays used today, called Hybritech, may give you a slightly higher reading than earlier tests. In order to compare different test results accurately, you may need to multiply your Hybritech score by 0.625."

"And," Paul added, "how they read your results depends on what part of the country you're in. Perhaps where you live they might take 0.1 as their standard. Currently in our area in the Northwest,

> Whenever possible, your PSA should be performed by the same lab and with the same method or assay used in previous tests to make sure the results can be compared. If your PSA does start to rise, don't panic. Ask questions such as whether there has been a change in the lab, because any changes in the lab or the methods used by the lab could affect the test results. Ejaculation can also raise the level of PSA in the blood.

less than 0.4 is as low as they're going to go. So there are big differences to be aware of. It also depends on the operator of the actual machine, their cleanliness, and whatnot."

"Adding to the confusion," said John, "is that now some doctors say that at a certain age you can go to 6 and be normal. Some are going as high as 0 to 10."

"Most of the doctors I've talked to," added Bud, "feel that 2.5 to 7.5 may be normal for a person who has their prostate after age 70. Before that age they're looking at 0 to 4."

So how often should you have your PSA tested? It depends on you and your individual case. You'll want to work closely with your health care provider in determining the best interval for you.

John and Virgil get tested every six months. "My doctor feels that if I want to go more than that, it's fine," John told us, "but he feels that because of my past history, six months is going to be OK."

"I was monthly and weekly for a while when my cancer was more active," Peter said, "and we were trying to change treatments. For example, when I first went to my oncologist, we were on weekly PSA tests for six weeks or so as he was trying different combinations and monitoring their effectiveness."

"And there's certainly more than the PSA numbers to keep track of," Paul explained. "When I go to my oncologist and I have a blood test, it's all-encompassing. He has a stack of different measurements—the white cell count, the red cell count, all the different things that help in determining my overall health condition—like is my liver working?"

"I also get a complete blood count (CBC) and a basic chemistry profile (BCP) at least once a month," said Charlie. "My PSA is measured at least once a month and sometimes several times a month depending on my treatment."

Some men, like Don, are diagnosed with prostate cancer with extremely high PSAs—sometimes reaching into the thousands. Some clinics, however, stop measuring past a certain number, such as 1,500, because there is no additional information or special treatments that apply when the PSA level is that high. According to experts, it's also difficult to tell what an extremely high PSA really means. (Dr. Ralph Weinstein, Prostate Conference, Portland, Oregon, April 1997.)

"I figure my oncologist's job is to basically keep me alive long enough so I can die from something else," Paul wryly observed. "And I'm totally satisfied with it. The important thing to remember is that you and your doctor need to think about and monitor all these other things—not just your PSA. So it's important to think about what kind of doctor will best suit you. Am I getting an overall picture of my health? Do I need to see a urologist, an oncologist, an internist, or all of the above? Fortunately for me, my PSA is currently stabilized."

As you can see, living with prostate cancer brings its own unique brand of stress: PSA testing, dealing with the side effects of treatments, changing treatments, changing your lifestyle, reevaluating your life. The ramifications can send your sanity packing—if you let it. Half of us are retired, and that, according to Paul, has its advantages. "I'm very, very fortunate that I have enough money that I'm not under pressure to go to work," added Paul. "I've tried to take all the stressful things out of my life and that's helped a lot."

"De-stressing is so important," said Charlie. "I actually, physically, just let go. (Charlie demonstrated by throwing his arms up in the air.) What you're seeing, this body language, is what I practice. I don't care. I'm letting go. I'm not going to let it get to me. I'm not going to be bugged, disturbed, upset, put under stress by anything or anybody. *No* one is going to get to me. I pray a lot too. I've always been a religious person. I'm an old altar boy, and old alter boys are a pretty defined group."

Religion and spirituality. Like politics, it's a subject that sparks strong opinions and provocative discussions. So obviously, for this group, it was a natural topic to tackle.

---

### Damaged Bone Marrow

If prostate cancer spreads to the bone it can affect your bone marrow. The bone marrow makes red cells that carry oxygen in the body, white cells that fight infection, and platelets that help clot blood. Any of these cells can be affected if the bone marrow has cancer in it. It is not unusual for your blood counts to go down as blood-producing tissues are replaced by cancer cells. If this happens, you may feel weak and tired. Your blood counts will be monitored, and if they are low, you will be told what type of precautions or treatments, if any, you may need to take.

---

We all agreed that everyone needs to find purpose and meaning in life. How we each achieve them is unique.

"I met a black minister and his wife, Carl and Mary Lou Williams," Charlie continued. "They have changed my life more than any two people that I know. One day Mary Lou stood in my driveway two inches from me and she threw up her hands and said, 'Charlie, you have to let go of that Rotary, let go of those other organizations, let go' (and she enumerated a list of things in which I was involved). It really got to me and I realized that with this disease, it had to be my number-one priority. I keep working on that. It's difficult to focus so intensely on just one area, but I keep improving and it's essential to my survival."

"That's why I call Carl and Mary Lou my 'God people.' They are so determined that religious healing can cure me that they keep trying to drag me to all these places and meet all these people they believe can help me. They feel very strongly about it, and in fact, we often pray together on my front lawn. And they have given me an outlook on life that I wish I could convince everybody to recognize and practice—namely, don't let the world or people get to you. In other words, you don't give out any crud, and nobody can give any crud back to you. It's just like a rod. It enables you to avoid control from other people. Throw the damn control rod away. Once you do that forever, you let go!"

"Can't hurt, that's for sure," said John. "It's definitely not invasive therapy!"

"Bernie Siegel, in his books," added Virgil, "gives a lot of personal accounts of people who've been considered terminally ill, but

When you're diagnosed with cancer, your life changes in many ways. Some people find that turning to religious or spiritual beliefs may help them cope. Others may feel angry and question their beliefs. Both reactions are normal.

because of their spirituality, their outlook on life, the treatment and the consultations they've received, they've recovered and the medical world is totally amazed. They have no explanation for it."

"I've got a great faith in God," said Bud, "and look upon prostate cancer as a challenge. In fact, I always say that life's not filled with problems, it's filled with challenges. I feel that if He or She's got a good reason for me to stick around, that's my job to keep going. I always say to people, you have to keep your attitude on high altitude. I would hope everybody who has cancer wakes up every morning and goes to bed every night and looks in the mirror and says, 'Hey, I'm going to beat this!'"

"I second that, Bud," said Don, "and I also think the good Lord thinks I've got a few more horses to shoe."

"Don, you're going to heaven in that big carriage in the sky," quipped John.

"I have to agree and disagree a bit with the conversation so far," Virgil told us. "I have the same kind of Catholic upbringing that Charlie and Bud had, but I kind of went astray from it a bit. We talk about the almighty and omnipotent God, and sometimes I feel that God is a practical joker—playing with us. I feel that I've seen too many good people have bad things happen to them and that makes me wonder, where is the fairness? Where is the justice? There's a test and we overcome it, but like I said, I feel that I've had enough character building in my life. I don't need to keep proving it. At some point, when do all the Hail Marys and all the rosaries add up? It should be like frequent-flyer points—you deserve to get a free ticket.

"I believe in God, but I find that my belief in God has gone past the traditional Catholic mode. I feel very comfortable going into a synagogue, into an Episcopal church, into a Buddhist temple, and talking to God. I feel just as comfortable walking down the street and having a religious experience. I think, probably, the thing that was important to me was to find God in myself. Too often we forget that we're made in His image. I'm very spiritual, and I believe in a

God. I just sometimes would like to know what's the plan and where are we going with all this. The old saying is He'll never give you more than you can bear. Well, you know, there's a debate behind that, and I have to question it sometimes."

"I am an agnostic," began Manuel. "At least I am now. My wife and I had four years of theological training and finished a few months before I was diagnosed with prostate cancer. I was also sexually abused when I was five years old. I had to live with the fear that I wasn't a whole man for 45 years—for 45 years. At age 45, I confronted my problems. I was able to talk to my wife about it, and when I did I became a whole man. No sooner did I become a whole man than it was taken away from me. I became impotent after the radical prostatectomy. And I am pissed! I don't like it! Virgil talked about God being a practical joker. This is a supreme joke."

"I'm sorry to hear that, Manuel, because for me prayer is so important," answered John. "I don't care whom you pray to, prayer is important. I've got my 'general' [Rosalie] sitting over here, and when she found out I had prostate cancer, we had already lived through the heart attacks and everything else. She got prayer groups going, and they sure gave me a lift."

"You talk about a loving, caring God," responded Manuel. "I don't see it. I am sorry, I do not see it anywhere. We were told in theological training that it's a loving, caring God. Where is it? I do not see it. It's gone. I got screwed twice in life—castrated twice—and I will never recover from it."

"One of the big points in the New Testament," offered Charlie, "is there are many passages about the fact that Christ was a healer. He worked many miracles of healing. My 'God people' have brought the practice of the black church into my life bigtime. They have reminded me of these scriptural readings. They have reminded me that I have to have balance in my life. One of the things that a strong religious belief does is focus you away from all your petty little concerns, your little egocentric views of your own life and its own importance, and put it in a different perspective. It also reinforces it with the fact that there's another being of great power who cares about you, and you can bring balance to your life, as acupuncture, for example, brings balance to the body. A belief in a religious position and a supreme being is extremely important for those who do have a religious belief. Just speaking for myself, it's absolutely central to my plan to beat this disease, and I want to remind you

Whether you are in the process of strengthening or reevaluating your spiritual beliefs, you might want to try the following:

- Take time regularly to meditate or pray in ways that are meaningful to you. These practices can create calm and stability in difficult times.
- Read spiritual writings such as the Bible, Koran, or Bhagavad Gita. Delving into sacred texts can put you in touch with long traditions of wisdom and give you a sense of connection with the holy. Recently published books on spirituality can also give new insights. (See, for example, *Care of the Soul* by Thomas Moore and *When Bad Things Happen to Good People* by Harold Kushner.)
- Seek the support of others. You might begin an ongoing dialogue with your clergyperson or counselor or join a group for meditation, prayer, and support. Discuss painful or distressing feelings with them. Don't try to handle this alone.
- Retreat to spiritual spaces or natural settings. Listening to fine music and appreciating beautiful surroundings can help you feel connected to a greater whole.
- Keep a journal to express your feelings, thoughts, and memories. It can contribute to your process of self-discovery and spiritual development.
- Pay attention to moments of beauty, peace, love, and hope. Share them with others and capture them for recall during times of distress.

(Courtesy of Cancer Care, Inc., 1180 Avenue of the Americas, 2nd Floor, New York, NY 10036–3602, 212–302–2400.)

that I have the worst case here. No one has ever survived, to the best of my knowledge, systemic, refractory, metastasized cancer. And I am going to try to be the first one."

"The thing is," said Virgil, "what's going to save us, ultimately—whether or not we acknowledge there's a force out there bigger than us—I think we have to find the bigger force in ourselves. God helps those who help themselves."

"I'm in a different position than any of you," said Peter. "I have no religious background or training. I respect all the world religions that I'm aware of and what they teach as far as how to live. And I respect all of you for whatever your beliefs are, but I don't feel the need to have the same thing. I'm not an atheist. I might be an agnostic. And as far as how I cope, religion has never been a part of my coping mechanism for anything my whole life."

"I have just one comment," said Rosalie. "There's a big difference between religion and spirituality. We all know people who go to church and profess to be whatever, and you can be deeply spiritual and stand on Mt. Shasta, or on the Matterhorn, or by the ocean, or you can be out in a meadow. If something in you responds to a universal wisdom and you feel uplifted, that's wonderful. You're right, Virgil, the kingdom of God lies within, and this is the seat of the healing mechanism. There's a book called *Spontaneous Healing* by Dr. Andrew Weil that says people have to get in touch with their spiritual center. It has nothing to do with an organized religion."

"I'm very comfortable being a spiritual person," responded Peter. "I've been out walking at 5:30 in the morning. I can talk to my God then. I'm not sure who or what I'm talking to, but that's my coping mechanism. I do have spiritual experiences and am rewarded by them, but I do not have any specific organized religious connections."

"My God lives within me," summed up Bob. "It's a very personal thing to each and every one of us, and I would not judge lest I be judged. But I do have a spirituality in dealing with my problem, and how I cope is with my God that lives within me."

"The only way I cope," said Manuel, "is I reach out to others. I am obsessive about reaching somebody who has a problem similar to mine. That's how I find fulfillment."

In fact, that's how a lot of us find peace and fulfillment—talking to other men with prostate cancer, helping to educate and acting as advocates. It's a way for us to give back.

"Don touches a lot of people," Lynne told us. "And he's never been afraid to talk to people, but he talks to them in a different way, with more understanding, now than he ever was able to before. He always wondered how come I've always been such a support person to others. I'm a lay counselor and for a lot of years it's always kind of bugged him—how can I spend all that time helping people and talking to them on the phone and never get paid and 'blah, blah, blah.' Don has never been understanding about that—until now. In fact, guess who's spending more time on the phone helping people now?

"And it doesn't have to be prostate cancer," Lynne pointed out. "My dad has been diagnosed with bladder cancer. Before, Don had always shied away from these situations and would have been the last to go visit someone. When my dad was diagnosed, however, he couldn't get over to him fast enough. He walked in, took his hand, and said, 'Brother, I'm here for you.'"

"Manuel's the same way," said Mary. "Every time Manuel hears about anybody that he knows who's been diagnosed, he's immediately on the telephone talking to him. I think if you know anybody in your circle of friends, or if they know somebody who has prostate cancer, I think one thing we can do as a friend is say, 'Let my husband talk to you.' Just be aware of people who have been diagnosed, whether they're single or married, and talk to them."

In fact, all of us talk to a lot of people in the course of our work. Charlie, for example, is the chairman of the Legal Action Committee for PAACT (LAC-PAACT), and John is one of the directors of US TOO.

"Because I work at US TOO International," said John, "I'm heavily involved with prostate cancer, but there's a big difference when you're involved with other people's problems. You become not only a survivor, but you're trying to help somebody. So between working on our house, my work at US TOO, and some other things Rosalie and I have going—life goes on. The key is I'm not going to sit down, look at the wall, and say, 'What have you done to me, God? Why me?' Why not me? I'm encouraged. I'm optimistic that in time a solution will be found, so I don't worry about it. I'm concerned; but worry? No."

Bud spends a lot of his time helping other people, too. "I give talks all over the country, and people call and thank me or they ask, 'What can we do to say thank you?' And I say, 'Come to my eightieth birthday party five or six years from now—when we have a prostate cancer–free society.'"

"The bottom line is that we have to involve the community and the family totally in this," said Virgil. "Prostate cancer is not just an individual's problem. It's a family problem, it's a corporate problem, and it *is* society's problem. It's a ripple effect, and you have to do everything that you can to try and stop the damage or at least minimize it. One of the things that I did at the little hospital not too far from where I live is that we set up a primary care center out in the community so that people could come in, get checked and screened

## The Physical Benefits of Laughter

Just as emotions like grief and anger can chip away at your immune system, laughter may help give it a boost and provide all kinds of other physical benefits as well.

- Laughter increases the number of natural killer cells, which seek out and destroy cancer cells.
- Laughter lowers the level of stress hormones in the blood.
- Laughter temporarily lowers blood pressure.
- Laughter reduces pain.
- Laughter reduces muscle tension, and that in turn eases psychological tension.
- Laughter exercises heart muscles—especially important for senior citizens or patients who have a difficult time walking or are confined to bed.
- Laughter triggers a breathing pattern that can have respiratory benefits by lowering the amount of residual air in the lungs and replacing it with oxygen-rich air.
- Laughter helps you maintain a positive attitude, and that helps your body fight disease.

on a variety of issues. But we also tried to educate the kids in school on the health issues that can impact their parents. So you get a little girl who says, 'Daddy, I just saw something about prostate cancer. When's the last time you had a PSA?' That's the kind of pressure that will have an effect—if all of a sudden it's personal and you get your family saying, 'Daddy, I don't want you to die.' That's an imperative for me. Get out all the false images you have of yourself and find the reality. Part of that for me is using the Internet, which was a major educational tool for me, and pass on my knowledge to others. I've created a website that's designed for people to find out about the disease, and I've started publishing a couple of how-to manuals. So I've kind of dedicated my life to making a new life for myself. These are things that are really important to me. Everyone needs to find what's important to them, cling to that, and make it a life goal."

We all survive and cope in different ways—by helping others; through spirituality; by refocusing on relationships, families, favorite pastimes, work. You, too, will find your own "normalcy," as

Peter put it. At the beginning of this chapter, we talked about the good times we had here at this retreat. In fact, not a session went by when we didn't erupt into laughter at some point. It's very true that prostate cancer is a serious subject and living with it brings all sorts of frustrations, disappointments, and tears. But we're also adamant about one thing: You have to laugh at yourself—at least once in a while. According to John, "A good laugh really reduces everything down. It takes the pressure off."

"Celebrating my impotency," said Manuel, "namely, joking about myself, has been extremely good for me. Just celebrate it. Get it out in the open."

"We both joke around about it," said Mary. "It's very healthy, and it's a great tension reliever. When we're both getting uptight about things, interjecting humor is a great tension reliever."

Peter added a medical note. "Your blood pressure goes down, too, so laughter is really good for you."

"I also think it's critical to be able to laugh at yourself," said Charlie. "In fact, I think it's a measure of your psychological temperature. People who can't laugh—particularly at themselves—really need help."

"I wholeheartedly agree," said Bud. "I found that I could laugh at myself when I'd make a bad mistake out on the tennis courts. When I should have put one away, I'd walk to the back, chuckling all the way. It's great to laugh at your own mistakes because it doesn't bother other people, and it really lets you know you can make plenty of them and still laugh and come through this thing. All these things really make a difference."

"There are a couple of books out that talk about the best cure for a lot of diseases is laughter and how people have been cured with laughter," said Virgil.

"Like Norman Cousins," answered Rosalie. "He was told he was terminal and he spent hours watching the Marx Brothers and the Three Stooges and that kind of thing. What I learned from that is the immune system is energized if you simply keep the corners of your mouth lifted. I started telling this to people, and I said on top of that, if you walk around with what looks like a half-smile on your face, people start to smile at you. Then you really smile back and the more you smile, the more the good juices flow. A smile is a circle of love. You can never give it away. It keeps coming back to you. Keep smiling and laughing and hugging and holding hands because that's got to be one of the most therapeutic things you can do for each other."

Speaking of jokes, this one is courtesy of Don: "Somebody says your fly is open—well, so what? Anything that can't get up—can't get out!"

So as we live with prostate cancer day by day—are we survivors, patients, or both? "Until I start looking at that grass from the bottom up, I'm going to be a survivor," said John. "Just listening to our conversations here, we are all survivors. I don't care what treatment we're taking. We're patients because we're still looking for alternate methods and better therapies. Yes, I am a patient. I'm on hormonal medicine. I go in and get my shot, and I'm also on Chinese herbs. I may not be cured, but by golly, I'm a survivor."

"I second that," said Paul. "If you're still alive one day after you're diagnosed, you're a survivor."

Charlie countered with this argument. "I think we're really talking semantics. I'm a patient—a fighting, positive patient. My problem with the term survivor is that if it hasn't been cured, the only way we'll know whether we've survived is when we die of something else. Patient sounds like a weak term, and I think that's why we don't like it. I'm the only person here who feels as if I'm a patient, but I'm a very aggressive, empowered, active patient. So I guess I share with John the duality of the role."

"The first thing I tell people," said John, "is that I'm a survivor. I still have prostate cancer, and we're still looking for that magic pill somewhere down the line, but I am a survivor."

"My desire is to live," said Bud, "number one. And my second desire is to spread education like every one of us is doing. That's really our job."

"Words aren't really that important to me," Peter told us. "I don't feel strongly that I'm a patient or a survivor. I do feel I'm surviving—to me somehow there's a difference. If you're putting me to the wall, I'd rather pick surviving than survivor. Because clearly, I am."

Clearly we all are.

As Charlie summed things up, "I think if you do not consider cancer an absolute enemy that's out to destroy you, your family, everything that you live for and love, then you're crazy. And I think if you don't treat cancer as something to be destroyed, that you'll lose a lot of your effectiveness in your fight against this disease. And if you don't have that attitude, then I think you're virtually giving up."

## Reflections on My Father

### by Lisa M. Russ (Charlie's daughter)

Dad thinks he has to convince us that he has cancer, and maybe we do need convincing. I hear what he tells me about the metastasis and the fluctuations in his PSA, but it's difficult to accept that Dad is sick when he is racing from his computer to the filing cabinets or to any other place he wants to be, just as he always has. One of his many funny characteristics is that even if the room is only eight feet long, he runs, not walks, to the other side to get something.

One thing that makes the cancer real is the elaborate structure of drugs that Dad takes. When he shows me the complicated drug schedule which he is on and the lineup of all these different and expensive medications, I'm impressed with the seriousness of his disease. At the same time, it seems as though doctors really don't know that much about it and just keep throwing drugs at it. Sometimes I get angry for Dad and Mom not only having to deal with the disease itself, but having to pay extravagant amounts for what are shots in the dark. In the ordinary world where I can get lulled into believing that there are solutions for most problems, cancer is a mystery and it's difficult to accept that no one has the answer.

Except on certain religious questions that are inherent mysteries, or on anything mechanical or related to some household appliance, Dad has always had the answers. In order to fight his cancer and the frustrating lack of answers, Dad has taken on some tangible enemies such as insurance companies, Medicare and the American Urological Association, and has become a formidable foe. He has armed himself with truckloads of information about his disease, rallied support

*(continues)*

"I also believe that if you focus heavily on your quality of life, do things, stay active in your work or other activities you're interested in, stay focused on your family, hang in there, keep fighting, keep your religious faith—for those who have it—you just live life and see what happens."

*(continued)*

from cancer patients all over the country and attacks the injustices of the system, which is where he is at his very best. If the subject matter weren't cancer, I would almost say he was having a ball.

Dad will never give up any fight, which is one of the most admirable and exasperating things about him. "I'm fighting a war!" he told me one Fourth of July on the front porch after we had held a small demonstration on my parents' front lawn during the Leawood City Parade. After the usual string of grade school bands, little girls with batons and Corvettes driven by various Leawood residents, the mayor sailed by, sitting up on the back seat of a convertible. Unlike the rest of the parade route, she received no smiles and waves when she passed by our house. She wanted to put a big unnecessary sidewalk on our street where practically no one is ever seen on foot. There we stood with our signs, "NO BIG GOVERNMENT," with Dad looking very serious holding his sign very close to himself so that you could only see his eyes. I maintained the family solidarity and did not smile or wave at the mayor.

Given my 36 years of experience with Dad, I'm not surprised that he has taken charge of his disease and organized his troops. He used to call the five of us kids "the troops." He's not superhuman, though. I know that he has to continually overcome anxiety and sometimes hopelessness, and that this is the biggest battle of all. We've had many conversations about his cancer, and I know that I've helped at times, and not at others. I still cannot believe that with my Dad's powerful will that he can't conquer this maddening unknown. He spent many years as a labor lawyer for Montgomery Ward and always told us that the only thing that could kill him was a Sears truck. That kind of statement is the essence of my Dad.

# 6

# *Sex, Love, and Intimacy*

*I don't know if you can understand the feeling of rage. It's like you're given a cookie. You taste the cookie, and all of a sudden it's taken away from you. And it's a very filthy joke. I don't like it. I don't have to like it.*

—Manuel Vazquez

When you're diagnosed with prostate cancer, there's one phrase that can immediately turn your blood cold: "Mr. ———, there's a possibility of impotence from the treatment."

Although intellectually you may know that treatment is necessary for your survival, the thought of being impotent can bring a devastating dimension to the emotional trauma that you're already dealing with.

"I recall," Manuel told us, "that just prior to treatment, I was told I was probably going to lose my sexuality; that regardless of the treatment, one way or the other, the risk was there. And eventually, it actually happened. I recall just crying—just crying like a baby—what am I going to do? It was totally devastating to me."

As Virgil explained it, "So much is tied into the notion of our penis ruling our lives—that if we can't get it up, we can't perform, and therefore, we don't have a function. We don't understand the image of giving, of loving, of self-esteem, that says we're more than just a 'swinging dick,' pardon the expression, ladies, but it's the only way I can really get it across. That's what's been ingrained in us for so long."

**143**

---

*Impotence.*   Impotence is one of the most feared side effects from the treatment of prostate cancer. It is defined as the inability to get and keep an erection adequate for sexual intercourse. Many of the treatments can also cause a loss of libido, or interest in sex.

---

It's an attitude that's been ingrained and sometimes shellacked—making a tough exterior that's difficult, but perhaps not impossible, to crack. As we tried to convey in Chapter 5, a diagnosis of prostate cancer served as a wake-up call to many of us, an opportunity to really understand who we were and what we wanted out of life. And with this disease your resolve and your self-image will be sorely tested!

"I think we men wrongly equate sexual functioning with manliness," Bob told us. "And we feel that if we can't function sexually, then we've lost our manliness. Right, wrong, or indifferent, that's a fact. We like to take pride in our sexual prowess."

"That doesn't always hold true," Peter countered. "I'm impotent and I miss the sexual interaction with my wife, but I really don't feel less manly. Those feelings may have been challenged to the point that I felt like I was losing it, but I'm quite comfortable now."

As John pointed out, "We're all different." And that is certainly true. Your comfort zone regarding your sexuality may be quite different from the guy's next door. "There's also a certain segment of the male population that doesn't put as much emphasis on sexual relationships as others do," added John.

"Oh—I put a lot of emphasis on it!" responded Peter. "I'm just saying that in having lost that, somehow it's still OK. I was very active sexually and enjoyed great pleasure and passion with my wife. I think, though, that my understanding has grown as I've gone through surgery, radiation, and some experimental treatments. And I didn't totally lose my sexual ability immediately after my radical. I had one nerve bundle removed, so my sexual ability was impaired. Then the radiation impaired it more, and the chemicals did more. It's been an extended period of adjustment. Plus, I'm also a diabetic and hypertensive and take drugs for both those conditions, so at this point, I don't think there's much chance of getting back my normal sexual function."

"Abnormal's good!" quipped Virgil.

---

### Impotence from Surgery

Two tiny nerve bundles straddle each side of the prostate. These nerve bundles transmit messages to the penis and are responsible for erections. If the nerves are injured or cut, messages can't get to the penis to allow blood to enter. If the cancer is confined within the prostate, your surgeon, depending on his or her skill and the technique used, can usually preserve one or both bundles. Some men can retain potency with only one nerve bundle intact. You can still have normal sensation, sex drive, and orgasm even if both bundles are damaged or removed.

---

Abnormal, normal, or none at all—your sex life will change. Your life will change. And it doesn't matter who you are—dealing with those changes will be a physical and mental challenge.

"We had a psychologist who used to come to the US TOO International meetings," Rosalie told us. "He had prostate cancer and spoke to the group several times. He had a fabulous marital relationship with his wife and was passionate in every part of his being. He got up in front of the group and told us that when he was diagnosed with prostate cancer, he went into their bedroom and cried to the point where he said, 'I'm glad I grew up in a family of Italian ancestry where we were taught that it was OK to cry.'"

"This gentleman that Rosalie is talking about had an orchiectomy," continued John. "From that time on, I don't think he could really take the fact that he had the orchiectomy. It was downhill from there on, and he didn't live but a few months after that. He just could not take the fact that the orchiectomy was something where he lost body parts."

Manuel asked, "Do you think he willed himself to die?"

"Yes," answered John. "I think that's exactly what happened to him."

"I need to make a comment here," said Paul. "Whether we are medically castrated with hormones or through an orchiectomy, like I was, the physical effects of stopping the testosterone are the same, and I don't know how somebody could cause their early death because of that feeling. Nobody could be a worse pessimist than me, so I think it's important that we know the actual castration part is the same."

---

## More on Bilateral Orchiectomy (castration)

Castration works almost immediately to reduce the body's amount of testosterone. Within three hours after a bilateral orchiectomy, testosterone levels drop to the "castrate range," which is often considered the gold standard when monitoring the effectiveness of hormonal therapy. Castration causes a loss of libido, or sex drive, and the inability to have an erection. (P. C. Walsh, J. F. Worthington. *The Prostate.* Baltimore, MD: Johns Hopkins University Press, 1995.)

For many men, the main disadvantages to having a bilateral orchiectomy are the psychological and cosmetic side effects. In one study, the majority of men (78 percent) elected for drug therapy over a bilateral orchiectomy. (B. R. Cassileth, M. S. Soloway, N. J. Vogelzang, et al. Patients' choice of treatment in stage D prostate cancer. *Urology* 33, Suppl. 5 [1997]:57–59.)

To ease the psychological trauma, some surgeons use a technique called a "subcapsular orchiectomy." The surgeon opens the lining to the testicles and removes only the testosterone-producing parts of the testicles. The empty shell is placed back into the scrotum so that nothing looks different. Some surgeons do not use this technique because they feel they may leave some testosterone-producing cells behind.

---

"All I can say is, that man's attitude changed," continued John. "He quit coming to meetings, and when he finally came back to our meetings he was a different man. He would sit there and stare into space."

"Maybe he was mentally castrated?" suggested Manuel. "I don't know if I could ever have an orchiectomy because it would go to the very core of me. I think I would probably rather die."

It's clear that whatever treatment you choose, sexual impotence can require a tough emotional adjustment even if the impotence is temporary. For some that adjustment is the equivalent of grieving over a loss—for you and your partner. That's why it's important to recognize the loss as serious and allow yourself time to grieve.

"Grief takes different people different lengths of time," said Phyllis. "Some people lose someone very dear to them and they're able to heal themselves and go on maybe six months or a year later. Other people go years and years. They still feel that loss, and they learn how to cope with life, but they still grieve. Let's face it. Almost everybody here is going to have to go through a grieving period over what they've lost. It's just a matter of how long it takes each person. We're all different."

"All of us have gone through this," emphasized Paul, "regardless of the treatment we've chosen. We've all had to face up to it sometime, and then you've got to make a transition. You just can't ignore the problem. Some of us are able to do it without pain, some of us with pain, but it's a transition. I have a real psychological problem because my world—our world—is so sexually oriented and it was a tremendous change for me. All of a sudden I don't even think about sex. I see a beautiful woman—nothing. It's a huge change."

"Paul was always a very sexual person," said Phyllis. "Sex was a very big, important part of his life. So I think of all the things he has sacrificed, or however you want to say it, sex is probably the one thing he grieves over more than anything else."

"I get a kick out of John," Rosalie told us. "He'll say, 'The most gorgeous girls in the world with the biggest boobs could walk by me, stripped naked, and it wouldn't even interest me.' He just doesn't have a sexual drive anymore."

"Fortunately," said John, "Rosalie is taking a very strong, supportive interest in prostate cancer and all it entails, and we work as a team. She understands what my feelings are, and I understand what her feelings are. And we work things out, and I think we have a very happy marriage. What more can I ask?"

"One of the things that's been a great outlet for me," said Paul, "is doing physical things, like working on some kind of building project, so I can put my mind to that kind of thing and release physical and mental energy towards that. The biggest thing I have in my life is a loving wife who takes care of me and supports me. Sexually, I don't know quite what to do for her, because I have no sexual desires or anything, but it's a problem we've been able to cope with, I guess."

"As far as our relationship goes, I don't think it's changed," Phyllis elaborated. "By that I mean, we still have a lot of closeness. We've known each other so long. We've been married 46 years, and so we've been together since we were teenagers. There's still a lot of closeness and touching. So I don't think we've pulled apart at all, in the sexual way, it's just without the act itself. I miss it, and he does, of course, but life goes on. And when you really come right down to it, the one sex act itself is a very small part of a day. The rest of the day you're still functioning in your normal routine. It's something that was a big, important part of our life before, but we've just learned to go around it.'"

"You just have to go off in a different direction," concluded Paul. "And fill the sexual void with something else."

But for some men, that is not easily done. For Manuel, the sexual void in his life has become a festering wound.

"I am a very angry person," he began. "I am impotent. I have lost my sexuality. And the impact of that is an anger that is eating me up. It's almost like a joke. I had a dysfunctional marriage for 25 years, and all of a sudden I had an ideal relationship with my second wife, Mary; ten years of bliss. And then I lose my sexuality. It's a loss that I cannot recover from, and the anger is so overpowering that sometimes I cannot control it.

"One thing I did is I shut myself off from my wife," Manuel continued. "All of a sudden, I would not even talk to her. We had a very good relationship where we could discuss the most intimate things. And at one point Mary said, 'You are pulling apart from me. You're just literally pulling apart from me. I can bear the lack of sex, but I cannot bear the being apart.' We finally put the finger on the wound; we knew what it was."

"Looking back, that was one of the few times in our marriage when he was not really able to open up to me," Mary told us. "All he did was withdraw. He didn't want to talk to me at all. That's what was so difficult for me, because we've always talked to each other about everything—the good stuff and the garbage. One of the things we did before we got married was, we laid out all our garbage on the table. He said, 'This is who I am,' and I said, 'OK, this is who I am.' I just knew it couldn't go on like this, and I couldn't tolerate that. It certainly wasn't doing him any good either. I put my foot down and said, 'You've got to do something!'"

"The problem," Manuel continued, "was if we had any degree of intimacy, I felt it had to ultimately lead to sex, which couldn't be. So I thought I shouldn't do anything, and that's why I shut myself down from all intimacy, completely. This has been devastating to me—totally devastating. And it probably has to do with my self-image as a man, feeling less than a man."

"He would get so depressed," remembered Mary. "He would go to a support group once a month—and that was really good for him. But then a week later, he'd start getting depressed. And then the next week, he'd get a little more depressed. Then the next week, he got *really* depressed."

"It got so bad that at one point I began getting drunk," continued Manuel. "I had never gotten drunk in my life, and all of a sudden, I was stone drunk. On the weekends, I could not bear the thought of having lost my sexuality because I felt that it was not only my sexuality I was losing—I was losing my relationship with my wife. I was suddenly afraid that I was losing my wife and my marriage was gone. We had a foolproof relationship, a very satisfactory relationship, and it was gone.

"I need to tell you that I was sexually abused when I was five years old, and I had to live with the fear that I wasn't a whole man for 45 years. At age 45, I confronted my problems and was able to talk to my wife about it. And when I did, I became a whole man. No sooner did I become a whole man than it was taken away from me. And I am pissed! Somebody had played a dirty trick on me. It was the supreme joke. It is an overpowering anger that I feel, and even right now, I feel the anger eating me up inside.

"And I began to really lose it. I began seeing the world as an evil place of randomness. I thought about suicide. I really thought I was finished. Finally, it got to the point that Mary said, 'You and I have got to talk.' She said, 'I can deal with no sex, but I can't deal with this. It's got to stop.'"

"I told him that he couldn't go on like this," Mary said, and 'I don't intend to go on like this. So you better go and get some outside help. Because this is not an avenue towards a solution for anything.'"

"Mary really forced me to go into therapy," Manuel continued. "I began going on my own for a couple of months. We've also gone a couple of times together and had some individual sessions."

"And I think it's helped a lot," added Mary. "The psychologist told us about some exercises we could do. You go for a week, and you caress and touch each other, give each other backrubs and everything, but no genital touching. Then you go through another week, which is that plus genital touching, and you work forward from that. So we are in the process of that. Well, we're supposed to be, but Manuel always wants to 'finish off the job.' And I'll say, 'But honey, we're really not supposed to do this.' So we try to have a sense of humor about it."

*Closure*

Even if you are unable to have an erection after a radical prostatec-tomy, you may still have normal penile sensation and sex drive and may be able to achieve orgasm through direct, physical stimulation. However, after a radical, there's usually no ejaculate or fluid because the prostate and seminal vesicles are gone. The feeling of orgasm, though, should be the same as during normal ejaculation.

Dry ejaculation can also happen if a certain muscular valve in your bladder neck is damaged during surgery or during a TUR for BPH. If this happens, semen can travel backward into the bladder during or-gasm instead of traveling out of the body through the urethra. This is also called retrograde ejaculation.

If you are on hormonal therapy and stop, your potency and libido should return to "normal." However, it does take time for the effects of the hormones to wear off.

"You were afraid," Virgil told Manuel, "just as I was afraid, that because we couldn't get it up, we were going to lose our women; that somebody else was going to come along who was bigger, stronger, whatever, and walk away with them. Fortunately, my head softened up enough that I was able to understand it. You've got a hell of a wonderful woman, and the fact that you are allowing a lot of crap that happened before to block you from being able to accept that love and to give all the love that you've got doesn't make sense. You've got so much inside of you that is important and beneficial and good and caring that to allow it to be summed up in four inches just doesn't make sense. It just doesn't make sense."

This raised a whole other issue: "One of the things we didn't talk about as the result of a radical prostatectomy is that you lose inches." Virgil had a way of getting our attention. "Fortunately, there was enough to start with, so it wasn't so bad," he joked.

"But seriously, the fact is that we're more than that. We're much more than that."

It's hard to describe not only the mood, the feelings, and the emo-tions that poured out from Manuel and Mary at the retreat but the responses that poured in from all of us—feelings of understanding and words of advice offered not in criticism but in support.

"I think it's counterproductive to harbor so much hate and bitter-ness and anger because of what's happened to you," said Bob. "I think that's really not conducive to being as healthy as you can possibly be. It just doesn't help you at all. If you can purge yourself of that, somehow, and focus, as Virgil was saying, on the positive and on your lovely wife and what you can give her and what she can give you and how supportive she is of you—you've got to consider yourself very grateful and very blessed to still have that."

"If he can purge himself," noted Paul, "and that's a big IF."

"But you'd be more cheated, Manuel, if you were in that little coffin," continued Bob. "That would be the end of it. I'm sure Mary's much happier to have you the way you are than laid out in a six-foot pine box."

"That's what I told him," said Mary. "He was ready to just let it all go, not to have the surgery. He said, 'I'm just going to die the way I am, all in one piece.' I said, 'Well, I can live without you, but it would be a lot more fun to have you around—in whatever shape.' We all lose different things."

"Manuel, you've given so much to all of us here," offered Virgil. "Maybe you need to start giving to yourself."

"I would like to say one thing," said Bud. "I was a life insurance man for more than 38 years. I paid many a death claim, among friends as well as strangers. The greatest thing the widows suffered was the loss of companionship, and if anything I could say here would help, it's that even though you may not have the sex life, the fact that you've got each other, to have someone to go to dinner with, to wake up in the morning with, somebody beside you—you may look at this day and count your blessings and say, 'Hey, maybe it's not as bad as I thought it was.' You look at the good side versus being in a coffin. It might change your whole view on life."

"Let me also tell you about two very sad experiences," Mary offered. "There are two elderly single gentlemen who are acquaintances of Manuel's. They felt that they could never, ever have a relationship again with a woman because of their problems. One is impotent, and the other man is both impotent and incontinent. I just told them, 'If you only knew how many women there are out there that would love to have a companion and have a relationship with someone, it would boggle your mind. There's probably more than 20 women out there for every man. It just broke my heart to hear them say that. I just felt so bad because that's not true. That's not the way it is."

Sex and love. Let's get one thing straight about those two little words. They may be constantly linked, but they do not share a com-

mon definition. That's a concept that crystallizes if you are diagnosed with prostate cancer.

"One of the things that has come through to me with stunning
impact is that men confuse sex and love," explained Rosalie. "Sexual intercourse does not have to follow a display of affection. This is
a very common male hang-up. A woman loves to be caressed,
hugged, or touched; hold her hand, stroke her hair, stroke her body,
and let her stroke yours. When I hear men thinking that just because
they can't have an erection, their love life is over?! This is tragic because they're confusing one thing with another. I think I shocked
some gentlemen one time. I said, 'You know what, gentlemen? A lot
of the ladies are relieved if you don't bother them anymore because
you weren't that great in bed to start out with. They're tired of fak-
ing orgasms. Now, they just want to look forward to your companionship, your intelligence, and your warmth, and that does not require penile interference, shall we say?' The point is one thing
doesn't have to go with the other. I had one woman tell me that she
agreed with me 100 percent. She said, 'As long as my husband's
alive and can hold my hand, that's all the love I need from him. Just
to have his presence.' So if men can get past this idea that their love
life is over just because they cannot have intercourse anymore, that's
going to be a major breakthrough.

"John and I are living a celibate existence, but that doesn't bother
me because we express love in many ways toward one another. It's
very important to have the laying on of hands, this tactile contact,
and again, there are all kinds of wonderful little ways that you can
convey love and affection. That's one of the things we've really tried
to help people understand."

"I always felt that if you were affectionate," Manuel told us,
"then you have to end up having sex. And for me, sex could not be.
So it was a no-win situation. I remember telling Mary that she was
free to leave me because I was impotent."

"And that hurt—that hurt real bad," answered Mary.

"Of course it hurt," said Rosalie. "It means that you don't really
understand this tremendously deep interconnection that the two of
you have spiritually and intellectually. It doesn't depend on a sexual
act at all."

"You're right," said Charlie. "I don't think the relationship between husband and wife has to deteriorate. I think there's an opportunity for it to be different, but different doesn't mean less. It is dif-

ferent, and in many ways there are things that occur in the relationship that are intellectual, that are spiritual, that are emotional, that are really much better, and that has been true in my case."

In fact, that has probably been true in most of the marriages represented at the retreat. All of us agreed that communication and mutual support become paramount when coping with sexual difficulties and the changes they have forced on our lives.

As John put it, "The key to all this is openness. You've got to be able to be open with your wife. You've got to have an understanding. You've got to talk plainly about your feelings. With my background, it was no matter how much it hurts—don't say a word. And Rosalie has been able to worm a lot of my worries out of me. She has that ability."

"Lynne was very supportive of me, too, and Rosalie said it all," began Don. "My wife told me all those things when I was diagnosed—about not needing the sex. She was really supportive. But the impact on me was still really devastating—just knowing that you had to go on this hormone therapy was something. I'm not used to being on drugs of any kind, any medication, nothing."

"Don was without sexual ability for about nine months," Lynne continued. "And it did bother him. I did try and tell him that it didn't matter, but until we came here, I didn't think he really heard me. And at first, if we were affectionate, he did pull away, somewhat. But he also knew that he probably wasn't going to be impotent for the rest of his life because he was probably going to go off the combination therapy at some point."

"I was on combination for about 12 months," Don remembered. "And when I went off of it, everything came back within 30 days or less. But the entire experience was devastating to me. That's why I'm here—to try and help anybody else get through this."

"He may be impotent again at some time," Lynne told us. "He may have to go back on CHT. I'm perfectly fine with it. However we live our lives, that's the way it will be. And I think he's beginning to believe that now, yes, it's all right with me and it can be all right with him, too."

Bud had a different perspective on sex, love, and intimacy. "After listening to you fellas who were diagnosed at a younger age, I see some advantage of my being 68 when my cancer was found. My wife and I had been married many, many years. We had an excellent sex life, and I don't say that because we had ten children—five sons and

## Treatments for Impotence

If you are having impotence problems, the first thing you'll want to do is talk with your doctor and your significant other—and have patience. Depending on your age, stage of disease, and treatment, it can take a few weeks or a few years for potency to return: If the nerve bundles were damaged during surgery or radiation, they take a long time to heal. Most men, however, find that their erections gradually improve over time. Impotence can be treated with surgical and non-surgical methods:

- Vacuum devices—A vacuum device is an airtight plastic tube that is placed temporarily around the penis. An attached pump is activated to withdraw the air, creating a vacuum around the penis. This vacuum causes blood to flow into the penis, which causes an erection. An elastic ring, which acts like a rubber band, is then placed around the base of the penis. This traps the blood and allows you to keep the erection intact. The device should be left on for no more than 30 minutes, so that blood can circulate again.

  Because there's no fresh blood circulating through the penis, it becomes cooler to the touch after a period of time. This is objectionable to some patients and their partners. (S. Marks, M.D. *Prostate and Cancer.* Tucson: Fisher Books, 1995, 249)
- Penile self-injections—Drugs such as papaverine, phentolamine, and prostaglandin E-1 can produce erections by causing the arteries to open and fill the penis with blood. At the same time, the drugs cause the veins to close—so the blood remains in the penis. The drugs are injected into the penis with tiny needles and produce normal erections lasting from 30 minutes to a couple of hours.

*(continues)*

five daughters. My wife had a breast removed 22 years ago because of breast cancer, and when I was diagnosed with prostate cancer, she was with me every step of the way. How much more can you say to be thankful for? I had such a good relationship that this hasn't affected our life together at all. We just take one day at a time."

Taking one day at a time is a philosophy shared. "I'm impotent from the cryotherapy," Derek told us. (Freezing the prostate can damage the nerves.) "However, I'm also starting to have sexual feelings and a partial erection, and I'm starting to think that maybe this

*(continued)*

It's important for your doctor to determine the lowest possible dose of drugs to minimize the risk of side effects. If the injection is too strong, it can sometimes produce an erection that won't go away (priapism) and may require medical attention to have it reversed. Other side effects can include scarring at the injection site, infection, tiny blood clots, pain after injection, and a lowering of blood pressure, which can cause problems for men with heart disease.

- Urethral medications—New devices such as Muse® (Medicated Urethral System Erection) are available for the treatment of impotence. The drug alprostadil is delivered via a suppository into the urethra, where it is absorbed through the wall into the surrounding erectile tissue. It increases blood flow into the tissue to achieve an erection.
- Oral medications—There are new oral agents under investigation by the FDA, including oral phentolamine and sildenafil (Viagra®). Sildenafil increases blood flow to the penis and in studies has helped 70 percent of men achieve erections. (Sildenafil was approved by the FDA in April 1998 and is available by prescription.)
- Penile implants or prostheses (bendable, mechanical, inflatable, and multicomponent inflatable)—These devices are surgically implanted into the penis through an incision in the scrotum. Some of the devices have pumps that are self-contained inside the cylinder; others have a separate pump that is placed in the scrotum and a reservoir that is placed in the abdomen. One note of caution: Implants should be considered permanent and are often used as a last resort. If you do have the implant removed, erections won't be possible even with other treatment options such as vacuum devices or injections.

is going to come back. So I'm optimistic. I don't have complete loss. The nerve system is there. I tried the vacuum devices, which did no good. I also tried the injections, but they didn't work well either—the erection wasn't any good. But I'm optimistic, and my significant other and I are able to talk things out."

"I also tried the injections and the vacuum devices," said Peter, "and they both worked, but neither was satisfactory for me. And then, of course, I went on the Lupron, and that killed the libido, so there was no need to use either one or try other things."

"I'm almost two years post-op," Manuel told us, "and in the last three months, the erections are starting to come back, which is consistent with what the doctors told me. I've tried the vacuum device. That didn't work. I tried the injection, but that didn't work either. The pain was so horrifying, I thought I was going to go crazy. It lasted for about two or three hours, and it was worse than anything I'd ever experienced.

"I finally ended up going to an impotency specialist," Manuel continued. "They ran what they call Doppler studies to see if my hydraulics were OK. He told me that I had no problem with my hydraulics. Both my nerve bundles were spared and all along my doctor said if it was going to come back, it would come back in two years. This was just at the edge of two years. The twenty-fourth of this month is my second year, and I do get erections every night, but they're not sufficient for penetration. But even if my erections are poor, that tells me one thing. The nerve bundles are working. There's something there. So that gives me some degree of hope."

"He does have erections when we're affectionate with each other," Mary added. "We've both been through a lot of frustrations with all this. And like Manuel said, we've tried the vacuum device and the injections, and sometimes these things have worked, sometimes they haven't worked. When they have worked, it hasn't been 'good enough.' It was good enough for me, but it wasn't good enough for him."

"You can find alternatives, too," said Manuel. "But if you come from a background like I did, growing up as a Roman Catholic, it's different. The church teaches us as children that alternatives are nasty. These teachings are internalized, and I feel nasty when I go to alternatives. I had to deal with that, and yes, we do alternatives, but I still feel like a nasty person. It's another burden because it's so ingrained in my development. It has really screwed me up. And I'm no longer a practicing Catholic. I still feel damned if I do and damned if I don't.

"The way I look at it right now," Manuel concluded, "is if my erections don't fully come back, then my only shot is an implant. But I'm fully aware that an implant is final. It's out there forever, and I don't want to go lightly into something that I cannot reverse. In the meantime, I do the best I can. I am very lucky that my wife is extremely supportive. Ultimately she told me one day, 'I'm more interested in security than I am in sex. Even though I enjoy sex very much, my security is more important, and your companionship is more important.' And we both broke down and cried, but I am still very angry, and that anger will not go away. The rage is internal. I've told you that I was a person of faith, but I've lost my faith. I see the world as an evil, random place. What has helped for me is channeling my anger into helping other people. I probably would have destroyed myself if I hadn't done that. The anger was so overpowering, I just had to go and reach out. That's how I find purpose for the 'joke' that was played on me."

"You can alter your response to what is happening," Charlie offered. "You can either take it in a negative way and have anger or take it in a positive way, as a challenge, and say, 'I'm going to beat it or deal with it.' I think anger is negative energy."

"Maybe for you, Charlie," said Virgil. "Maybe that's the way you deal with it. But I think anger is a healthy situation. It allows a catharsis at times, maybe to vent what shouldn't be left inside of you. Maybe you can come out and vent it in terms of elocution or whatever. Maybe Manuel needs anger to get the rage out of him. So I don't think that we should say that anger is a negative thing. It may be negative for you, but maybe not for him. We should be able to say OK. That's how he's dealing with it."

"Let me put it this way," Manuel explained. "The anger I cannot control. It's there. And I don't make any excuses for it. I didn't do anything to get cancer—maybe I did, I don't know, but the anger is there and I have to come to terms with it. I still channel it by reaching out to others. That's the only way I can find some purpose. This is what the dynamic is. This is what happened to me. I have to help somebody else. It has become almost obsessive. I try to reach somebody and I'm positive with that person, but I will never, never sugarcoat—to anyone. I will tell the person clearly what may happen to him."

"One thing we don't want to do here," observed Peter, "and maybe Manuel is feeling this, is pick on him, and say, 'Why the hell don't you change?' What I hear, and I hope you're hearing, Manuel, is that all of us are encouraging you to do whatever you can to try to get over this hump of feeling that you're in this terrible position. Maybe some of our stories of how we've gotten past this and how we're much happier where we are now and have better spousal relationships than we had—maybe these comments can encourage you to try and find your way to do the same thing."

"I am angry," responded Manuel, "but I also see all of you, and my heart reaches out to you. You are in another stage, where I may be sometime down the line. And when I see that I think, 'Damn— why am I so angry?' I should not be angry, but I cannot help it. Fortunately, I know I've been blessed with the ability to verbalize, but this is the first time, here at the retreat, that I've been able to express in public how I felt without sugarcoating, and without any concern for how somebody else feels. Obviously, I was enraged when I was telling you my story, but being able to verbalize it and the impact of saying it in public has helped me a lot—and I thank you for that."

And that is our wish for all of you—that our experiences help *you* to sort through your own feelings during this transition period in your life, and, as Peter put it, "encourage you to find your own way."

## Nighttide II

### by Cindy Stults (Peter's wife)

On the bed
he lies on his left side
right arm reaching
behind his knee
left arm beneath his head
in the quiet of our room
I sit in the rocking chair
the fan's gentle whir reminds me
of the soft sleep he must feel now.
His six foot frame
seems small on a king size bed,
but as I look at him in his drizzle slumber
I see his grey temples
warm against those high cheek-bones,
and his eyelids closed
like petals over an indigo bloom
I almost climb in next to his skin
his wide arms bear all the truth of his strength
while the hair upon them is kin to a young sheep
it's now I think of all those millions of cells
gathered inside this piece of art
"Billions of cells," the doctor says,
"millions are in the size of a pencil point;
billions in the diameter of a pencil,"
and he named it cancer.
rapid cancer.
It is now that the full beauty of his body
lying on the left side
comes into focus
and I lie close in to his skin.

# 7

# A Woman's Point of View

## THE WIVES' STORIES

*You have to be very patient, and you just have to keep loving them, and reinforcing the fact that you love them in whatever way that you can.*

—*Mary Vazquez*

Phyllis Georgeades, Rosalie Plosnich, Mary Vazquez, and Lynne Zank. We are the partners, the lovers, the confidants—the wives. You've been hearing from us all along because this is our story, too, and we felt it was important that our thoughts and viewpoints were represented. That's why we came to this retreat—to complement our husbands' perspectives by offering our own. Four women and ten men. We held our own quite well, thank you.

We've all heard that a diagnosis of prostate cancer affects everyone in the family. To try and illustrate that fact, we've been talking as frankly and openly as possible, and we hope that our comments are helping you to understand some of the ramifications of living with this disease. Not that we're experts in the human condition, but we have been experiencing prostate cancer right along with our husbands. We, like them, have weathered the hard knocks, been beaten up emotionally, shared their disappointments and joys. We share their anxiety as we wait, together, for the latest test results. And together, we have survived.

What's our secret? Perseverance, a little luck, and a lot of love on both ends.

Rosalie Plosnich is an architect. She and John have been married 30 years. "I couldn't put my finger on what was happening with John," began Rosalie. "But the quality of his life was starting to fade. I could see there was something happening to him, and I was concerned. I knew he was overdue for open heart surgery, but there was something else. Well, God works in mysterious ways. One day in June of '91, I couldn't sleep and the *Chicago Tribune* skidded against the door. I got up, got the paper, and it fell open to an article by an angry wife who had found out that her husband had advanced prostate cancer. He'd been having annual exams for 20 years, and he would always tell the doctor that his father and brother died of prostate cancer—even that he had to go to M. D. Anderson because he had another brother who was terminally ill with prostate cancer. She was furious because that's when she found out about what I later learned was the PSA test. She wrote to Ann Landers—and I never read Ann Landers—'Angry wife asks for people to find out about simple blood test.' So at 9:00 in the morning, I called John's cardiologist and said, 'I want an order for this test for John.' John's on blood thinners and he has to have blood drawn every month, so what's another vial of blood? And the cardiologist actually gave me a hard time. He said, 'What are you ditzing around with?' I said, 'Look, if you don't give me the test order, I'll get it from my OB/GYN or my internist, but I'm going to get it, and it would look better if it came from you.' I slapped the test order into John's hand. He got his PSA tested and the score was 182. The cardiologist nearly went into cardiac arrest!"

"I had known for six years that Don's urine stream was not quite right," began Lynne. "His nephew, whose father-in-law had died of prostate cancer, was his apprentice, and he told me that Don needed to be checked because *he* could hear Don's urine stream was not right. But as you know, Don was a workaholic and he didn't have time for such things, so it just didn't happen. Then, by chance he noticed in the paper an advertisement for an after-hours clinic that would do prostate checks. He decided to do it, then, because he wouldn't have to give up any work."

Mary Vazquez is the choirmaster at her church. "For us," said Mary, "I think it came down to the fact that it was time for me to have my yearly physical and mammogram, and I said to Manuel, 'Hey, I go in every year and get tested, and you haven't had a physical for ten years. Would you mind going in and having a physical done?' So I kind of nudged him a little bit."

Both Mary and Lynne have health care backgrounds. Mary is a licensed vocational nurse. Lynne is a registered nurse. So for both,

prostate cancer was not totally unsuspected. However, the reality of
the diagnosis was still a shock. "I can still remember the feelings of
fear that went through my body when we heard his PSA was over
2,000," recalled Lynne. "I knew that a PSA that high had to entail
bone metastases. Today, the doctors still can't believe that there was
no bone involvement."

"When I heard those words—prostate cancer—I was a little surprised," said Mary, "because everything about him seemed so
healthy. I kept thinking, well, the PSA was elevated, but there was
no palpable tumor or anything like that, so I kept thinking maybe it
was BPH. But there were also some other things about him that indicated to me that he might possibly be at risk. I had read many
years ago that there was a possibility of some connection between
vasectomy and prostate cancer. I knew he'd had a vasectomy. We
were also very concerned that there might be lymph node involvement or metastases at the time. And of course, we were anxious
about how we were going to face this. And there was a lot of worrying and caring because I didn't want him to suffer. You never want
anyone you love to have to go through any kind of either emotional
or physical suffering. And Manuel was also terribly concerned
about the future. At one time I think he even thought, 'Well, this is
it. I only have a little bit of time left. My time is up. My clock ran
out.' I can't really understand his anxiety because I'm not him. But I
also know that my level of anxiety was a little bit high. On the other
hand I knew he had youth on his side. I knew he was otherwise a
very healthy person. So that helped to subdue some of my fears, especially my fears of metastases. I knew he was only 55 and we
caught it early, so I was reassured by that."

Depending on your individual circumstances, a crisis can either
split up a relationship or cement it. For Lynne, drawing on her
strong faith was a cornerstone for survival—and the survival of her
marriage.

"Since 1986, I had made a conscious decision to give Don Zank
to God and let Him take care of Don, because I wasn't able to do it.
We had had problems with our marriage, but I was going to stick it
out. I wasn't going to divorce him, but I had given up emotionally in
our marriage. And I had already done a period of grieving.

"When this diagnosis of prostate cancer happened," continued
Lynne, "I wasn't surprised, but when they said his PSA was over
2,000—I was shocked about that! But I thought, 'Well, God, what-

ever you've got in store, show us. Get me through this, and we will get through it—dead or alive, we will get through it.' So I guess my biggest feeling was shock because of the height of the PSA. Resignation and faith were other strong feelings, too. But I was also afraid of what Don might do.

"Don always told me that if he ever got cancer he would blow his head off. And he meant it, and I knew he meant it. In fact, he threatened suicide many times in many different instances. That was one of the reasons I had done a lot of grieving. What was bothering him? Just life in general. He comes from an extremely dysfunctional family, and within the last few months he's done more talking about his father than he's ever done in the history of our marriage. And I've heard some things I've never heard before. So that was one of the things I was dealing with. When there would be a loud noise out in the barn, I would jump! I went looking for him a couple of times not really knowing what I would find—and expecting he could kill himself at any time. Now, today, I don't think he would, since he has made a profession to Christ. I don't think that suicide is still an option. So we've been through a lot."

Phyllis Georgeades is enjoying being a homemaker and grandmother. "It was very hard for me," remembers Phyllis. "We got the news over the phone that it was cancer. At the time we received this news we were struggling with the fact that his sister was dying from breast cancer. And she did die about three months later. So when I heard this, I thought, 'Oh no, this is it.' Of course it wasn't. And after about six months, we started connecting to various people and gathering more information over the Internet. During that time I was at every appointment he had with his doctor, and we discussed all his options together. But Paul did the research. I encouraged him, but he got himself to the computer and read the books. And I continued to encourage him to keep digging—keep going. I was involved in decisions inasmuch as whatever he felt comfortable doing, I felt it was something he should do—*if* it wasn't going to be dangerous or risky. I didn't want him to be a guinea pig."

"Since we only have one computer," Mary added, "Manuel did most of our research, too, but he kept me informed about what he was finding out. And I also tried to read up on some things, and I attended support group meetings when I could."

Working as a team is a recurring theme throughout this book. We can't stress enough how important it is to attend support group meetings with your husband, if your schedule permits, and to try to keep current with the latest information. Just be involved!

"Support them," said Lynne. "Allow them to make their choices. If you can offer suggestions, if you can encourage them to go to a support group, that's great. Some men are more willing to be encouraged by their wives. Others have to find their own way."

"It's always been amazing to me," Rosalie told us, "that when we go to the US TOO meetings, how important a supportive wife is to these men. In fact, I think that if a wife doesn't attend support group meetings and isn't involved, it can put the husband in harm's way."

"Rosalie and I have worked together on a number of projects," continued John. (We'll let John speak even though this is the wives' chapter.) "And we've worked together and separately on these projects. Rosie's a great reader—a very good detective. When she starts digging for things, forget it. She's going to find it. She'll go to the library; she'll make phone calls anywhere in the country to get information. By the time she gets through, you could almost call her "Doctor." She absorbs it, and I'm not just saying this because you're sitting next to me, dear. The key here is working together."

All of us would agree with that. And all of us have tried to be there for our husbands from the beginning. We also know that our efforts have been appreciated because Paul, John, Manuel, and Don have told us. In other words, we also need support from our husbands. Living with prostate cancer can be tough going for everyone, and without a base of mutual trust and understanding it can become intolerable.

As Rosalie put it, "No matter what happens to you, that's not important. What's important is your attitude and the way you accept and cope with it. Since the time of John's first heart attack, I made up my mind that if there was any way humanly possible, plus the power of a lot of prayer and hard work, I would try and keep him on his feet and going. I think I've helped keep him alive by sheer force of my will. And I know he knows I love him a lot."

We all love our husbands a lot, and we will all continue to cope with whatever this disease hurls our way.

"Before Paul was diagnosed with prostate cancer, he was a pretty moderate guy who lived life on an even keel," Phyllis told us. "He was always pretty controlled. Now, I find that he does sometimes lose control. I don't mean in a rage, but he may just start crying or something may be hysterical to him and he'll go on and on about

If your husband has prostate cancer, one of the things you might find yourself coping with is a change in your husband's moods. Feeling sad or depressed is one of the most common emotions faced by cancer patients. It's often described as having feelings of gloom, despair, and emptiness, feelings that can change day to day or hour to hour. These mood swings can also be caused by hormonal therapy.

it—just very strong emotions. I can describe it as an emotional pendulum: He can be extremely happy; then he can hit way down to the depths of despair—and in five minutes he'll be back up again. I think this is in part due to the cancer and the treatments and all the other hormonal differences in his life. He works hard with all the other parts of his treatment, so I'm hoping that somehow he'll be able to get his emotions under control."

Here at the retreat, Charlie and John are living with the most advanced cases of prostate cancer. "God willing, John and I will be married 30 years this year," Rosalie told us. "And when you live with somebody that long and go through all the medical problems we had on the cardiac side, you watch him like a hawk. John has a very high pain threshold. When he talks about discomfort, the rest of us would be screaming our heads off. And one thing I've noticed in recent years is that he's been talking about pain, so I know he's uncomfortable, and we'll be watching this very carefully."

You've already learned that a lot of our husbands are also carefully watching their diets. In fact, some of them have drastically changed their eating habits. That's a lifestyle change that definitely impacts other family members. It's affected some of our kitchens, too.

"My kitchen is still in transition," laughed Lynne. "I'm still moving things around, throwing certain cooking items away, cooking utensils I no longer use because I have so many new ones. This is still going on after three years. And I'm still continuing to change because it's a totally different way of cooking. I enjoy cooking. I enjoy exploring new ways, new recipes, especially creating really nutritional things, so it's definitely changed. And when we invite our children over to eat, they're not quite sure about all this, but they're also getting to really like some of the foods. Our son, who lives with us, is very cooperative."

If your husband is living with advanced prostate cancer, he may or may not be coping with pain. Prostate cancer most frequently spreads to the bone, and pain is one of the major symptoms. It can also be a major challenge of living with this disease. But remember, there are several effective treatments to manage pain, including chemotherapy and radiation, and there are always new therapies under development.

Every case of prostate cancer is unique. How you and your partner respond to and handle the many nuances of this disease and its treatment will be unique, too. Nowhere is this more apparent than in the sexual arena. Manuel and Mary have testified to that.

"Every human being is very complicated," said Mary. "I think in my husband's case, yes, he is very sexually frustrated because he's impotent. I also know he's very angry about it, but I think the anger partially stems from some other things in his life that he has not resolved yet. I think in his particular case that this is compounding the issue and making it more of a struggle for him. He did have the nerve-sparing technique on both sides, and fortunately, he's beginning to have physical indications that his potency is returning. It's been almost two years post-op, but his doctors told him it was going to be at least 18 months to two years before he regains his potency. He has erectile activity at night in his sleep. And he does have erections when we're affectionate with each other, but as soon as he thinks about approaching me, everything goes to pot. There's a lot of other complicated things going on behind the scenes here. And I think it has to do with the way he feels about himself as a person, too. He got downsized from his job. He's 57 years old and he doesn't have a livelihood to go to every day. I think that's very important for all of us. You've got to have something to look forward to each day.

"As far as I'm concerned," Mary continued, "I've been through a lot of frustration with this. As Manuel told you, we've tried the injections and the pump, which haven't worked to his satisfaction. I think he has to come to the acceptance, too, that things will never be exactly the same as they were before the surgery. He's not 20 or 30 or 40 or even 50. The body changes, and things slow down. As far as my feelings, I *have* gotten frustrated when things didn't work out. I've gotten very sad for him because I know how horribly disappointed he is, and I know it must be horribly humiliating for a man to fail—that it's very uncomfortable. It's not a place where they want to be. I've gotten angry about it, saying, 'Why does it have to be this way?' especially for him because he's a person who needs to know that he's loved. I think that's another barrier he has to cross. He needs to recognize that he is a lovable human being just the way he is. Now I've gotten to the point where I'll be very cooperative with him. If he wants to experiment with something, that's fine with me because I love him, and I don't want him to think in any way that I would ever reject him for any reason."

"I've tried in many ways to reassure Don that his ability to perform sexually was not the most important part of life," Lynne told us, "and that this was not the most important part of loving. I think he's gradually learning this, but he's also glad that he's no longer impotent."

We talked about the difference between sex and affection in Chapter 6. But we feel that this is so important a topic that it needs to be revisited. Showing affection becomes a way of telling each other that you care, that you need and desire each other's companionship and physical closeness—that you want that person in your life.

And it works both ways.

"I've talked to a lot of people," said Rosalie, "and I've only talked to one woman who was bitter about her husband's impotence. She was furious, just very, very angry. She felt that her husband's impotence was enough for her to end the marriage. I said to her, 'What if you learned that you were going to have a double mastectomy?' She had a beautiful figure and she was also very vain, very selfish. I said, 'If you suddenly felt that you had to face your husband with the loss of your beautiful breasts, would you be hurt if he said, "I don't want you anymore because your breasts are gone"?' She never thought about it that way. I continued talking to her, saying, 'If you have self-esteem, if you believe you are worthwhile, that you're a wonderful person, you have a lot to offer, then losing two breasts is not going to change your soul or your inner child. If he would still have love for you and need for you, the loss of your breasts wouldn't mean anything to him, so why are you taking the reverse attitude?' And the saddest thing that we get are the calls from the men who want to divorce their wives because the men can't have intercourse anymore."

"I've just accepted the situation," Mary said. "Whatever will be, will be. This is where we are in our lives right now. And I have not given up hope yet because I think that once some of these other emotional barriers are crossed, things will get better. I have to admit that we do joke and kid around about it, which helps relieve the tension. Sometimes Manuel will say, 'Well, IT doesn't work anymore. I'm just a big failure—or THE THING is dead.' I'll tease him back about it. I'll say, 'You know, you're murmuring. You're like the people of Israel who went around murmuring all the time, and you need to look at what you have here. Don't murmur.' We've laughed about it and we've cried about it—lots of times. I've talked to him over and over again about the fact that I need affection, and now I'll just tell him, 'I don't want sex. I just want you to hold me. I just want to sit with you. I want you to put your arms around me. I need a hug.'

"Most of the time, though, I still have to be the initiator," Mary continued. "A lot of times he still will not reach out to me affectionately because he thinks he's inadequate, because he can't get an erection and have intercourse. But now, sometimes, he will reach out to me, just reach over and touch my hand or something, and it makes me feel wonderful when he does that!"

"We've also learned to replace the sex with other things and other signs of affection," Phyllis told us. "There's more holding, more hugging—just spending more time together."

"I think we just need to tell our husbands that it's OK to be impotent," Lynne concluded. "That you did not marry them for their penis and that there are many other parts of them that you want to be a part of your life."

One thing we have stressed throughout this book is the importance of communication and talking about the issues that surround this disease, issues that can affect your marriage and even threaten its existence. Lynne says, "You need to keep saying the 'right' things and supporting your husband whether they seem to be listening and 'receiving' or not." And, as Mary has said, "in order to deal with anything, you have to talk about it." But for many men *and* women that is easier said than done.

"I want to relate to you an incident that happened to me very recently that really brought some things home to me," said Mary. "I'm normally very open. I talk very openly with my daughters, and I'm usually pretty open about what's going on in my life with my close friends. But a couple of months ago, I went in to have a mammogram. They called me back in and said the radiologist wanted to take a closer look. So they did some additional X rays on me. When I looked at those X rays with my doctor, I saw a spot on my breast. So I'm asking myself, 'What is this? There's no cancer in my family.' But I was anxious to get home and tell Manuel what was going on—but I could only tell him. I wanted to call my daughters and tell them. I wanted to call my prayer group at church and tell them to pray for me because I didn't know what was going on. But for some reason, I didn't want to tell anybody else. And I'm not usually like that. One of the reasons was fear. Maybe there was something there. And of course, I didn't want to upset my daughters until I knew something for certain. Anyway, there was nothing wrong. There was a spot, but there was nothing to worry about. But boy, did I understand right then and there what Manuel went through. It was WOW! Maybe that was a channeler, an avenue for me to get some little inkling of understanding. I can't explain why I didn't want to tell anybody, but I can certainly understand now what it must be like for someone to have that hanging over their head. It helped me to understand what it's like waiting to have a PSA. Every three months Manuel gets very anxious because he has to go and have the blood test again. My experience was a real eye-opener for me, and now I can really empathize a lot more."

More understanding, better communication, a change in values. In Chapter 6, our husbands talked about the changes prostate cancer had brought to their lives—and the 'good' that had come from this disease. We took that concept a step further and talked about the 'gifts' that prostate cancer had given us.

"I believe that God really has a plan for our lives," said Lynne, "and we can fight that plan or we can decide to look for good in everything. There's been more good in prostate cancer than anything that has ever happened to Don Zank. It has improved our relationship tremendously. He began to trust me, and that trust has just grown and grown. We've been married 34 years, and this might sound strange to people just hearing it, but prostate cancer has truly been a gift to our marriage, our life, our children's lives, and our family.

"Don is a different man. His personality has changed, and he's much easier to live with than before the cancer—much easier. He's much more understanding and patient with people. He's less judgmental. He's less perfectionistic. He realizes what's important in life and what isn't. And he's much more willing to talk about touchy details that he didn't want to be bothered with before. He hugs our children more and shows them more emotion and caring than he ever has before. He's still a workaholic, but he's trying to not let that rule his life."

"I can't get over that," commented Rosalie. "I held my arms out to Don and he came over and gave me this big hug! This is a man who before wouldn't hug?!"

"I told you he'd changed," said Lynne. "And these four days at the retreat have been wonderful. The first day and even the second day, Don told me and our kids, 'I'd rather fight Mike Tyson than go there. It would be over quicker!' But last night he wouldn't go fight Mike Tyson. He'd rather be here. It's been wonderful."

"Part of the 'gift' for us is in the spending time together," added Phyllis. "When Paul was diagnosed, he stopped working and retired, so that brought us together again. And I really think that is a gift that we're both enjoying. I keep laughingly saying that we're now joined at the hip because we hardly spend any time apart. I go into the bathroom and there's the dog, the cat, and Paul standing there! But it's been great."

"I think that my gift in all this," said Mary, "is that I am able to minister to other people who are going through serious illnesses or death. Sometimes all I do is sit there and hold someone's hand. But I think I am able to go and be with somebody else and be a comfort to them when they're going through something like this."

"I think that's one of the gifts for me, too," said Rosalie, "being able to help others through a crisis and be there for them in every way. But I also think that one of the gifts that prostate cancer has given all of us is that we were all brought here together. We would never have met each other if it wasn't for this so-called dread disease. If I wanted to put a title on this sojourn that we're having, it's a *celebration of life*. And for that John and I are both grateful."

We are all grateful for a lot of things. Prostate cancer, in theory, is not one of them. It is a terrible, heart-wrenching, life-threatening disease that we wish on no one, and we pray daily for a cure. But what has happened in our lives because of this disease is truly amazing. We have met people that have changed our lives, and we have changed the lives of others. We have changed ourselves. We hope we have helped others cope with this disease with our heartfelt experiences, support, and advice.

"Be patient," said Mary. "Be loving and go along with your husband if he wants to try something new. Go ahead—go for it! What may not work for somebody may work for someone else."

From Lynne: "Don't be intimidated by the doctors."

From Phyllis: "Ask questions."

And from Rosalie: "Never give up hope."

# 8

# *Money Talk*

INSURANCE AND FINANCES

*"Don't take no for an answer" seems to fit pretty well here.*
—Derek Workman

Just about the time you start adjusting to the fact that you have prostate cancer, you're faced with another challenge: dealing with your insurance company. If you're lucky, (1) you have insurance, (2) it's adequate, and (3) it covers whatever therapy you choose to have.

But even if you have a good health care policy, the treatments for prostate cancer can induce sticker shock. Just ask Don. "It was devastating," he remembers. "I had a $5,000 deductible policy. I was paying all my biopsies out of pocket at $100 each. Then I decided to go on combination hormonal therapy. At first, the assistant in the office wouldn't tell me what that cost. She just sat there and said, 'I can't believe what the price is. I hate to tell you.' 'Well, what is it?' I asked. She said, '$450 a shot.' Then the doctor came in and said, 'Sell it to him at my cost—$375.' Even so, when I started paying this out of my own pocket, I immediately began thinking about how many horses I had to shoe and how many I had to trim. It was really devastating to me."

So pull out your policy. You'll need to find out exactly what your health insurance covers and exactly what you'll be expected to pay, and that includes any complementary therapies. As Charlie says, "The first thing that should be done by anybody is to read their insurance policy very, very carefully and, if necessary, get a legal opinion on it. You'll also want to talk with your doctors and their office staff. They submit the claims in most cases and should know who pays for what therapies."

> *Insurance Cap.*    Do you know what your insurance cap is? A cap is
> the lifetime amount that your policy will cover for a specific illness,
> and it's a major issue for people with cancer. Every policy has a cap
> on it. Some pay up to $100,000. Some pay $500,000. Some up to
> $1 million. If you are nearing your cap and are able to change poli-
> cies because you're still working, you may want to try to find one
> that has a higher cap. You may also want to try to purchase a policy
> that is guaranteed renewable.

Even better advice, especially if you're reading this book and
haven't been diagnosed with prostate or any other type of cancer
but are concerned about the possibility, read your health insurance
policy carefully *now*. If it's not adequate and you have the option of
changing it or adding more coverage, you may want to consider doing just that!

"And read between the lines," added John. "You get an education
once you start reading policies. It's such fine print that if you're not
a lawyer or someone who does a lot of detailing, you're going to
miss something because you tend to start jumping around. Insurance is something all of us should be concerned with because in the
long run, we're all going to be involved one way or another."

As Paul put it, "I think the attitude to have is, whatever the cost,
I'm worth the money."

"That's all well and good," responded John, "if you've got the
money. "I think we're *all* worth it. But with some men we're talking
$1,500 for a three-month Lupron shot. They're not on Medicare
and they don't have insurance, and that's a lot of money! And if
they're on flutamide or Casodex, you're talking another $10 a pill
per day—times 30. Plus any other medication he might need!"

"When I had my first heart attack, my first bill was $88,000. It
was 55 pages long and that was only a partial. I've already gotten
over $400,000 in bills, between the prostate and the heart. I've got
pills that cost me $1.50 a day and some I take three times a day. If I
had to pay for it, my savings would be depleted rapidly."

You'll also want to keep tabs on Medicare: Know how it's currently
set up and keep abreast of any changes coming down the pike.

"Once you reach age 65, you should take both A and B of
Medicare," suggested John, "because from the doctor's standpoint

*Medicare.*   Medicare is a federal health insurance program for people 65 or older and certain disabled people. It is run by the Health Care Financing Administration of the U.S. Department of Health and Human Services.

There are two parts to the Medicare program:

- Hospital insurance (Part A) helps pay for inpatient hospital care, inpatient care in a skilled nursing facility, home health care, and hospice care. You are automatically covered under Part A when you enroll for Social Security. Part A has a large annual deductible and coinsurance, but most people do not have to pay premiums.
- Medical insurance (Part B) is voluntary and helps pay for doctors' services, outpatient hospital services, durable medical equipment, and a number of other medical services and supplies that are not covered by Part A. Part B has monthly premiums, deductibles, and coinsurance amounts that you must pay yourself or through coverage by another insurance plan. Premium, deductible, and coinsurance amounts are set each year based on formulas established by law.

Medicare provides basic protection against the cost of health care, but it will not pay all of your medical expenses. For example, Medicare will not pay for self-administered medications such as pills, or most long-term-care expenses. Medicare pays only if you receive the medication, such as an injection, in your doctor's office. If you disagree with a decision on the amount Medicare will pay on a claim or whether it will cover the service at all, you have the right to appeal.

Many private insurance companies sell supplemental (Medigap) insurance as well as separate long-term-care insurance. If you are nearing retirement age, you may want to think about signing up for a supplemental plan.

*Medicaid.*   Medicaid is health insurance for low-income and indigent people, individuals who are disabled, and certain groups of children. Services are operated by state governments under federal guidelines, and the benefits and conditions vary widely from state to state. To apply for coverage or to determine your eligibility, contact your state or local department of social services. You'll need to provide information about your income and assets.

*Health Maintenance Organization.* A health maintenance organization, or HMO, is a type of managed health care plan in which members pay a set fee to an organization. The HMO then provides health care through its approved doctors and other providers. In HMOs, a certain amount of money is allocated to your treatment. If the money isn't spent, the doctor and the organization keep it. Thus any money spent on treatments for patients is money out of the doctor's and the organization's pocket. Some believe that this system effectively holds down spiraling medical costs by removing the incentives for unnecessary tests and treatments and focusing on prevention instead. Others see it as a conflict of interest for the doctors.

One of the benefits of a managed-care program is that you do not have to file claims and out-of-pocket expenses are kept to a minimum. However, these plans can be restrictive, and you may find yourself limited to a select list of hospitals and doctors who may not have expertise in a particular treatment or procedure that you may want.

The federal Medicare program is currently experimenting with managed care. If you are enrolled in Part A and Part B, you are eligible to enroll in a Medicare-contracted HMO if there is one in your area. Medicare HMOs often provide more comprehensive coverage, sometimes at the same monthly fee as traditional Medicare.

on part B, you can't beat it. Sure you pay something on it each month, but it's worth it. Then get yourself a good supplemental policy. Blue Cross/Blue Shield is cheaper than AARP (American Association of Retired People), but I decided to sign up for AARP because I don't even see a bill anymore. Medicare automatically sends it to AARP. AARP automatically pays it. I used to spend hours each month going over bills, making sure they'd go to the right place, because a lot of doctors' offices would not take the assignment. I also signed up Rosalie on AARP. Between the two of us, I think it's about $260 a month. But again, it's worth it."

"I'm 65 years old and I *didn't* go on Medicare," said Peter, "because I'm a dependent on my wife's policy. My prescription drugs (excluding Lupron) cost about $1,000 a month, and they wouldn't be covered under Medicare. Through my wife's plan, I get them for about $35 a month. It made more sense for me to stay on her policy

The Department of Defense (DOD) and the National Cancer Institute (NCI) recently signed an Interagency Agreement that offers TRI-CARE/CHAMPUS-eligible patients access to NCI-sponsored clinical studies of new cancer treatments. TRICARE/CHAMPUS patients who enroll in any NCI-sponsored phase II or phase III treatment clinical study, nationwide, will have their medical care costs covered by CHAMPUS. This agreement represents an expansion of an earlier project launched in 1994 that authorized CHAMPUS to pay for CHAMPUS-eligible breast cancer patients participating in certain NCI phase III clinical studies.

Under the project all standard TRICARE/CHAMPUS rules, cost shares, and deductibles will apply for patients seeking care. TRI-CARE/CHAMPUS patients considering participation in an NCI-sponsored treatment must first have their physician confirm with PGBA CHAMPUS (DOD contractor designated as the national contact for physicians and patients) that the study meets the criteria of the demonstration project, and the physician must also receive preauthorization for evaluation of the patient. Physicians at the treatment institution will determine whether the patient is eligible for the NCI-sponsored study.

For more information call the NCI at 301–496–6404, PGBA CHAMPUS at 1–800–779–3060, or the NCI's Cancer Information Service (CIS) at 1–800–422–6237.

as her dependent. So I didn't suffer financially because most of my costs were, and are, covered."

Fortunately, most of us have good insurance policies. But when you have prostate cancer, not only are some of the treatments very expensive but a lot of the therapies are still considered alternative, experimental, investigational, or out of the mainstream, which translates to "coverage denied" by many insurance companies. Because of that, many of us have considerable out-of-pocket expenses.

For example, Charlie takes the drug Aredia® to help prevent bone loss caused by his metastatic cancer. Aredia® is FDA approved for hypercalcemia and bone metastasis caused by breast cancer, but it is not approved by the FDA for metastatic prostate cancer and is considered "off label" when used for this purpose. "It costs me $463 twice a month—all out of pocket," Charlie told us.

For others of us, the choice of treatment has meant resorting to a little creative thinking.

"After settling on seed implants, I thought, 'How am I going to pay for this?'" remembered Bob. "That was a bit of a problem because it was a nontraditional kind of treatment as opposed to a radical prostatectomy or external-beam radiation. My HMO, which was Kaiser, didn't cover it, and I wasn't old enough to get Medicare. So one of the reasons I decided to do watchful waiting was to get a year older—to qualify for Medicare." (Bob was comfortable with watchful waiting and believed it would not be harmful to his health.) "I celebrated a birthday and after about a year and a half, I withdrew from Kaiser, went into Medicare, and had Medicare pay for the treatment. The cost for my seed implants was about $22,000. I was out of pocket about 20 percent of that. So that's how I got my procedure paid for. When the open enrollment period allowed, I got back into Kaiser."

"I strongly believe," said Charlie, "that HMOs are out to restrict services and to restrict the payment for services by holding back treatment that you might need. And I think it's getting worse. Hospitals and other large organizations are also buying up doctors' practices and putting them on salary. And some doctors are quitting. The nature of health care in this country has already radically changed, and I think it will become even more difficult to get the kinds of services that we may need from health care providers."

"Even AARP is talking about converting to HMOs," observed John. "And I know darn well HMOs will opt for the cheapest therapy, and that's an orchiectomy."

"I belong to an HMO," said Paul, "and I've had my problems with insurance companies, namely that they didn't want to pay for my cryotherapy. I belong to a trade union, the International Brotherhood of Electrical Workers, and they elected not to pay. We were self-insured, and certainly we couldn't afford to pay for claims that weren't legitimate. But after the hospital sent me a bill for $16,000, I knew I had to do something. I had my doctor explain to them the details of cryosurgery, and after some letters from Lloyd Ney and PAACT explaining that the FDA neither approves nor rejects the medical procedure, my trade union finally saw the reasonability of cryotherapy and accepted and paid for the whole thing. They realized that this is a viable treatment and they went ahead and paid for it."

## Tips to Help You with Your Insurance Coverage

- Keep copies of all your insurance policies.
- Keep careful records of all covered expenses and claims. Make photocopies of all claims and correspondence with your insurer and doctor.
- Keep careful records of all telephone contacts with your insurer.
- File claims for all covered costs.
- Insist on written confirmations of any telephone agreements.
- If your claim is denied, first check for clerical errors and then look carefully at the reason given for denying coverage. Then file again. Ask your doctor to send the insurer additional information to verify the need for services.
- Make a written request for reconsideration and let your insurer know that you mean business. Be sure to include your policy and claim numbers.
- Be persistent. If the claim is still denied, file an appeal.

"I believe," said Charlie, "that if we, as health care consumers, do not unite to battle the insurance companies, the health care providers, and HMOs, we're going to get considerably less health care paid for under our insurance policies."

Charlie is the chairman of LAC-PAACT, the Legal Action Committee of PAACT, and has been a key player in successfully lobbying the American Urological Association to reverse its stand on cryotherapy and recognize it as no longer investigational.

"I will tell you that I have been fighting this issue at full speed with the AUA," Charlie told us, "and I will tell you that some doctors and insurance companies and Medicare are like unbroken horses—they do not want you on their back. And they will do everything to get your little body off their back. They will deny coverage to an unbelievable extent."

"We have to keep fighting," said John, "especially having gone through a lot of hard times with a lot of our support group members on cryotherapy. First, it was absolutely no! The insurance companies won't pay for it. Then, thanks to PAACT, who really jumped in on this issue, they started paying the hospital bills. Then Medicare finally started paying on it, but then the insurance compa-

> *Disability Insurance.*   This type of insurance can provide you with
> income if you are unable to work due to illness or long-term disabil-
> ity. These policies usually have a waiting period of at least one
> month. In some states, if you are employed, disability coverage is re-
> quired by the state and premiums are deducted from your wages. To
> find out if you are eligible, contact your local Social Security office.
> You can also purchase disability insurance through private insur-
> ance companies.

nies fought it for a while. Neither would pay the doctor's bill. It was
one battle after another. Even though a lot of us are 65 and over,
we're having one hard time."

"You could almost say that everything is experimental," John observed. "There's really nothing we do that isn't experimental because there isn't a cure. With regards to cryo, at least the insurance
companies are taking a second look. Some of our people have gotten their cryo paid, and that's a big relief."

Derek had some initial trouble getting the charges for his cryotherapy paid, but persistence and perhaps a little inconsistency on
the insurer's part prevailed. "I was covered by CHAMPUS at the
time. I'm a military retiree and I was under 65, so I was covered
by this military insurance until Medicare took over. I went to the
CHAMPUS office at the USAF hospital in Albuquerque and was
told that cryosurgery was *not* covered by CHAMPUS. This was after they had called the CHAMPUS headquarters office in Denver.
So I had a no from that source, and things seemed pretty final. But
I didn't give up—a lot of left hands don't know what the right
hands are doing. I figured that I would fight it later if I had to because I definitely didn't want radical surgery or external-beam radiation, which was way too scary for me. I decided that I wanted Dr.
Fred Lee of Crittenton Hospital in Rochester, Michigan, to do the
cryo, so I went up for a consultation and checked with the hospital
insurance office about coverage under CHAMPUS. They immediately said yes. They also called their regional CHAMPUS office to
confirm this and got another yes. Once I heard that, I said, 'Start
working on getting the job done.' Why they paid for my cryotherapy when the Denver headquarters said no I still don't understand."

---

### Prostate Cancer and Military Benefits

If you are a Vietnam veteran and have been diagnosed with prostate cancer, you are eligible to receive medical disability payments. In 1996, President Clinton added prostate cancer to a list of illnesses linked to Agent Orange for which the Department of Veterans Affairs will provide benefits. Agent Orange is the chemical defoliant widely used to clear jungle areas in Vietnam. Under government policy, all 2.6 million veterans who ever served in Vietnam and adjacent waters are assumed to have been exposed to the herbicide and do not have to prove exposure. The legislation, which is effective October 1, 1997, authorizes medical care, a stipend ranging from $200 to $1,200 per month based on the level of disability, and vocational training.

For more information contact your nearest VA medical center or regional office or call the VA's nationwide toll-free number: 1–800–827–1000.

---

"When I first went on hormonal therapy," Bud remembers, "my insurance company hadn't even heard about it because it was so new. Fortunately, I documented every month's prescription. My doctors dictated all the proceedings into a machine and five or six days later, I'd get a copy of exactly what happened and why. At the end of four months, I sent my insurance company the records and said, 'Here's what it is, these are the results we're getting, and would you take a look at it?' The insurance people had a meeting and said, 'Yes, we'll pay for it.' I also knew a lot of these people, which probably helped. Anyway, maybe I feel too optimistic on these things, but we *are* making headway on insurance coverage. And nobody should have to go without their therapy being paid for. We all need to be helping each other on this."

"I have a different problem from all you guys," Virgil said. "I'm still working and have the probability of working quite a few more years. So right now, I'm covered by my insurance. But what happens if I move to a new job? What about preexisting conditions?"

That depends. (See second box on p. 182)

"The bottom line," Charlie emphasized, "is that you have to *document* what you think is really needed—whether it's medicine, treat-

## Other Private Policies

There are also several private policies offered by some insurance companies. One policy provides a lump sum from $10,000 to $50,000 to the policyholder for any diagnosis of cancer. The money can be used to defray the costs of getting second opinions, out-of-pocket expenses not covered by your own health plan, or lost wages.

ment, or procedure—and you have to be empowered to fight it right to the wall. Insurance companies do not back off easily. In one of our cases, a wife documented every single inch of the denial for cryotherapy to the point where she had a file that was devastating, and when our lawyer was getting ready to go in with the final shot, the insurance company folded and agreed to pay for the cryo. So you can bluff them, but they don't bluff easily. And you've got to be prepared to go to bat against them."

And don't give up. You may have to go to the top of the organization to get what you want, but if you can justify your choice with strong documentation that a treatment has worked for others, you have a good chance of convincing even your managed-care plan to cover the procedure. It also helps to have your doctor on your side.

In 1996, President Clinton signed into law the Health Insurance Portability and Accountability Act. This bill will allow people to carry their insurance with them if they change jobs. However, insurance companies, especially managed-care companies, are undoubtedly looking at this very closely because they would be forced to cover high-risk patients. At this point, though, you are supposed to be able to take your insurance with you if you change jobs, and you cannot be denied a new policy.

Many states also have high-risk pools set up to sell insurance to residents with serious illnesses or preexisting conditions. The rates may be high, however, and the coverage may not be as good as other policies.

Medical costs that are not covered by insurance policies sometimes can be deducted from annual income before taxes. Examples might include mileage for trips to and from medical appointments and out-of-pocket costs for treatment, prescription drugs, or equipment.

# Pharmaceutical Companies' Indigent Drug Programs

We're listing only those companies that make products commonly used for the treatment of prostate cancer. However, almost every company has a similar program. If you are receiving a drug made by another company, get the phone number of their Medical Affairs Department from the *Physician's Desk Reference* (updated every year and available in bookstores and public libraries) and call the company directly. Ask for its Patient Assistance Program.

Hoechst Marion Roussel, Inc.
Patient Assistance Program
1–800–221–4025

Immunex Corporation
Patient Assistance Program
1–800–466–8639

Janssen Pharmaceutica
Provider/Physician Program
1–800–544–2987

Merck US Human Health
Patient Assistance Program
1–800–672–6372

Schering Plough Corporation
Commitment to Care
1–800–521–7157

TAP Pharmaceuticals
Care First Program
1–800–453–8438

Zeneca Pharmaceuticals
Assistant Programs
1–800–424–3727

Pharmaceutical Research &
Manufacturers of America
1100 15th Street NW
Washington, DC 20005
1–800–762–4636
1–800–862–4110

Patients who are ineligible for clinical studies and in an immediate medical crisis may be eligible for drugs that are waiting for FDA approval. Your physician must contact the Investigational New Drug Program and apply for an "emergency IND."

Single Patient Investigational New Drug Program
Food and Drug Administration
HF-12
Parklawn Building, Room 949
5600 Fishers Lane
Rockville, MD 20857
301–443–0104

## Suggestions for Finding Life Insurance

- Try to find a group plan. Employers and other organizations often offer group life insurance. Many credit card companies offer life insurance policies.
- Try to get a graded policy. Graded policies will return your premiums, plus a part of the face value of the policy, if you do not survive the first few years of being insured. If you live past the waiting period, your beneficiary will receive the full amount of the policy.
- If you are unable to get any other form of insurance, guaranteed-issue life insurance may be an option for you. With this type of policy, no questions are asked about health and no physical examination is required. The downside is the cost.
  Premiums are high, and you need to survive for a specified period of time (usually one to five years) before your beneficiaries can collect the face value of the policy.

With regard to cryotherapy, LAC-PAACT has developed a kit that contains Medicare judicial decisions ordering payment, documentation on the benefits of cryotherapy, and many important statistics. This documentation has resulted in a number of victories for patients. However, Medicare has recently (effective April 15, 1997) taken a "no coverage" position on cryotherapy and will no longer pay for procedures performed after that date. Many private insurance companies continue to pay for the procedure, but the cases are generally decided on an individual basis. As Charlie advises, "*Always* document, be patient, persistent, and never give up." For more information and to receive the LAC-PAACT kit, contact the offices of PAACT at 616–453–1477.

We talked earlier about the high cost of some of our prescriptions. Lupron®, for example, is one of the most common drugs prescribed to prostate cancer patients—and there is a great disparity in cost from doctor to doctor and pharmacy to pharmacy.

"One doctor charges $714 a shot for Lupron," said Charlie. "In addition to that, there's a second charge of roughly $35 just to receive the shot and additional charges on top of that. Another hospital sells it for under $500. Some discount drugstores charge around $420. It's all the same shot, and Medicare and insurance companies

*Viaticals.*    Viatical settlements are arrangements for people who have less than 24 months to live and who have active life insurance policies. Viatical settlements involve the cash sale of your life insurance policy to a third party. People who choose a viatical settlement generally receive about 60 percent or more of the face value of their policy immediately in return for signing the benefits over to the third party.

The Health Insurance Portability and Accountability Act contains a provision that allows people diagnosed with a terminal illness to get an accelerated death benefit (ADB) or a viatical settlement on their insurance policies without having to pay income tax on the proceeds. The new rules apply to proceeds received after December 31, 1996. The tax-free provision applies only to people whose purchasing company is licensed by the state in which they live, and the proceeds must be used for "costs incurred by the payee, for qualified long-term care services provided for the insured for such period."

If you wish to pursue a viatical, here are some guidelines:

- Talk to your health care providers about your life expectancy.
- Get at least five bids from competing viatical companies.
- Seek professional legal and financial advice from a tax attorney or an accountant. Know the tax consequences as well as how payments affect your eligibility for any other entitlement programs such as Medicaid.
- Weigh the immediate need for maintaining your standard of living and quality of life against the future needs of your dependents and beneficiaries.
- Ask your insurance company if you can sell only part of your policy.

*Life Estates.*    In some states, you can sell your home but continue to live in it for the balance of your life.

will pay all these prices and additional charges. Nobody is monitoring this. So when you wonder why the costs of health care are rising, it's these little built-in additional costs that are ridiculous."

"First of all," responded Bud, "that $714 is not a bargain. I check on this every six months. Some of the states are paying $375, which is all the doctors are charging. The normal charge is $425 if you go

---

## Other Options for Financial Assistance

*Patient Assistance Programs.* These are designed to help pay for drugs and are offered by most pharmaceutical manufacturers. To learn whether a specific drug might be available at reduced cost through such a program, talk with your health care providers or a medical social worker.

*Fund-Raising.* Many cancer patients find that friends, family, and community members are willing to help if they know about a difficult financial situation. You may want to contact your library for information on fund-raising.

*Transportation and Lodging Assistance.* There are nonprofit organizations that arrange free or reduced-cost air transportation for cancer patients going to and from treatment. Talk with a medical social worker or contact the Corporate Angel Network Program at 914–328–1313 or the National Patient Air Transport Hotline at 1–800–296–1217.

There are also organizations that provide lodging for patients and families receiving care away from home. Contact your treatment facility or the National Association of Hospital Hospitality Houses, Inc. at 1–800–542–9730.

*Community Service Organizations.* There are many agencies and volunteer organizations such as the Salvation Army, Lutheran Social Services, Jewish Social Services, Catholic Charities, and the Lions Club that may offer financial help. Check your local phone directory. Some churches and synagogues may also provide financial help and services to their members. And in some communities, the American Cancer Society or other cancer-specific nonprofit organizations offer modest financial aid for expenses such as transportation to doctor's offices, home care or child care, or other such necessary out-of-pocket expenses.

---

to the drugstore. Some patients go to the drugstore to buy the Lupron and pay a nurse $5 to give them the shot." (Don's wife is an RN and gave Don his shots.) "However, some doctors' clinics are trying to offset their drop in revenue from surgical fees—caused by the increased use of hormone therapy—by raising their costs of the drugs from $425 to $575. That gives them $150 extra every time the person comes in for a shot. Plus they throw in $35 to $50 for a doctor's call."

For more general insurance information contact your state insurance commissioner's office. Pamphlets and booklets include the following:

*Cancer: Your Job, Insurance and the Law.* American Cancer Society, 1989. Call 1–800–ACS–2345.

*Cancer Treatments Your Insurance Should Cover.* Association of Community Cancer Centers, 1991. Call 301–984–9496.

*Health Insurance and Cancer: What You Need to Know.* Kimberly J. Calder, M.P.S., and Karen Pollitz, M.P.P., 1998. Write or call National Coalition for Cancer Survivorship (NCCS), 1010 Wayne Avenue, 5th Floor, Silver Spring, MD 20910, 301–650–8868.

*A Consumer's Guide to Health Insurance: How to Understand Your Policy's Coverage and Challenge Claim Denials.* R. A. Peterson, n.d. Write or call Center for Public Representation, 121 South Pinckney Street, Madison, WI 53703, 608–251–4008.

Additional insurance resources:

Health Care Financing
Administration
(HCFA)/Medicare Issues
U.S. Department of Health
and Human Services
7500 Security Blvd.
Baltimore, MD 21244–1850
1–800–638–6833, 1–800–772–1213

National Insurance Consumer
Helpline
1001 Pennsylvania Avenue NW
Washington, DC 20004
1–800–942–4242

"A word of caution here," said John. "If you're on Medicare and you go out and buy this shot and pay $375, you may pay for it. Medicare will not pay for any type of medication not administered in the doctor's office, clinic, or hospital."

"In Michigan," said Lynne, "Blue Cross has to insure you. And even with Don's high PSA and everything else, they started paying $750 for the CHT the first month. They wouldn't pay the other surgical costs for six months, but they did pay for the medicine."

Now that we had our pet peeves and grievances on the table, we also talked practicalities. How can you beat the high cost of therapy?

"If we take a very practical look at this thing," said Bud, "the only way we'll ever really beat this is through our state legislatures and the federal government. One of the biggest lobbies in just about every state is the insurance business. We don't have the money combined that the insurance companies have. There has to be some fundamental reform."

"I think that's one way," said Charlie, "but I'm an activist, and that way is *not* easy. It takes a lot of money and time. One way is to take advantage of the fact that companies like Drug Emporium, for example, are in competition and, because of their volume and big purchases, are able to make drugs available at much lower prices. So a much easier way is to shop around for the lowest price. It's not a question of who makes it but who sells it. You go to the place where you can buy it the cheapest, just as you'd shop around for an automobile or a pair of shoes or any other commodity."

"Some drug companies," added Bud, "have compassionate-use programs and 800 patient-assistance numbers that you can call if you don't have insurance and can't afford a particular drug."

"And you don't have to be completely destitute," said Virgil. "In some cases, because of the cost of the treatment, some patients have been able to get at least part of their costs absorbed. Also, the U.S. Senate has, as part of its Department of Aging, an office that will work with constituents of either party in finding ways to cover whatever treatment is needed, be it drug therapy or anything else."

(For more information call the U.S. Senate Department on Aging at 202–224–5364 or 202–224–1467.)

Paul had some final tongue-in-cheek advice: "Have a lot of money and a good insurance policy!"

That includes life insurance. Getting life insurance after a diagnosis of cancer can be challenging, if not downright impossible. When you apply for life insurance, your medical history will be scrutinized in great detail. However, even if your recent health history has not been good, there are legitimate ways you can still get life insurance.

Although there continues to be health care reform movements in this country, many believe that the real revolution in health care is going to happen in cancer care. Perhaps the cancer community, patients, and health care providers can work together toward a model that lies somewhere between managed care and private insurance—where costs are contained but everyone gets the treatment they need, want, and deserve.

In some ways, Don was able to beat the system. "Before Don went in to have his PSA," Lynne told us, "he knew and felt that something was wrong, so he purchased another $100,000 worth of insurance and set up a really good plan. And he was right."

Sometimes intuition pays off, too.

# 9

# *Recurrence*

## STRATEGIES FOR SURVIVAL

*There are psychological benefits of having something to look for-ward to. For example if someone asks you, "What's your plan for the future?"—it's nice to be able to say, "Well, if this doesn't work, I can go on to this next therapy."*
—*Paul Georgeades*

Anyone who has squared off against cancer knows that his or her life has been affected in a profound way—in a way that's often im-possible to convey to others. Maybe one way to express this feeling is simply to say that an intruder entered our bodies and permanently violated our well-being. "A diagnosis," says Manuel, "is an event maker in your life. You become a teenager, then an adult. You get married, sometimes divorced, and all those events change your life. Prostate cancer also impacts and changes your life forever."

That's because even if you are one of the lucky ones who de-tected the disease early and it was confined to the prostate, and even if your treatment was "successful," the threat of recurrence, psycho-logical or otherwise, is always there for you and your family.

"Do I worry about it? It's in the back of my mind," Virgil told us. "I'm certainly not looking for it to return, but I realize the potential is there."

"I have already decided in my mind that it's probably going to come back," Manuel told us. "And the reason I do that is because if it comes back, I'll be prepared. I don't know if that's a pessimistic or a realistic attitude."

That depends on whom you talk to, and maybe the stage at which that person was diagnosed. According to Bob and Virgil, Manuel's view is pessimistic. "If you are realistic," Virgil explained, "you deal with the fact that today, I *don't* have prostate cancer, but I realize that maybe in ten years I will have it, and I'll deal with it then. But if you put the seed of potential in there, you put the seed of reality that says, 'I'm going to get it.' Maybe in your mind you don't want it, but if you put it in there and say it's going to come back, then you're giving it a life. You've got to deny it a life."

"The reason I think it's pessimistic," said Bob, "is I think that it tends to cloud the enjoyment of everyday life that you have right now. In my case, I try not to think about it. Now, I'm living every day like it's my last, and I'm enjoying every bit of it."

"I'm enjoying every bit of life, too," said Manuel. "I stop and smell the flowers because I may not be here in the next few years."

Regardless of our differing philosophies, we would all agree that simply realizing the potential of recurrence, no matter what your current stage, is probably a smart thing to do. That doesn't mean you dwell on the possibility or necessarily assume that there *will* be a recurrence but that recognizing the possibility spurs you to be prepared.

"In my situation," Peter explained, "I certainly don't want to say I'm anticipating it, because that would cloud my day-to-day existence, too, but I can't rule it out. I think what I would like to know, every day and every week, is what am I going to do *if* it recurs? That's my task now, and if I were to critique my performance, I'd have to say that I don't think I've done it adequately yet. One of the things I'm working on is trying to build my book of options and then, of course, keep changing and updating it as new treatments and therapies come out. In other words, this won't be a static list of options. Hopefully, it will change and improve as time goes by."

"For me," said Manuel, "realizing the potential prepares me for the eventuality that it might happen. Then, at that point, I will not be devastated. When I got my first abnormal PSA reading, I tried to tell myself I didn't have cancer. There was no history of cancer in my family. Even after my second PSA, which was even higher, it still didn't hit me. I went through the biopsy just simply to get the doctor off my back. I remember seeing the six biopsy cores on the table and thinking, 'No—I do *not* have cancer.' And then, the fourth day after the procedure, I got the call from my doctor saying, 'I want you to call me *today!*' My world caved in. It was total devastation. I had

*Primary Tumor Site.*   The primary tumor site is the location where a malignancy starts, such as the prostate. Sometimes cells from this tumor can break away and travel to other parts of the body through the bloodstream or the lymph system. These migrating cells create a secondary tumor. When this happens the cancer is said to have metastasized.

*Bone Metastasis.*   Bone metastasis is the spread of cancer to the ribs, the pelvis, and the spinal column, common with prostate cancer. Specifically, the cancer grows inside the bone marrow, where growth of new bone occurs. This can cause a variety of problems, including pain, anemia, hypercalcemia (too much calcium in the bloodstream), bone fractures, and spinal cord compression. In more advanced cases, prostate cancer can spread to the lungs, the liver, and (rarely) to the brain.

the rug pulled out from under my feet, and I don't ever want that to happen again!"

It's called self-preservation. As we talked about in Chapter 5, all of us have our PSAs regularly tested. But according to Bob, that doesn't mean he's constantly worrying about the return of his cancer. He's just playing it smart.

"There's no point in being stupid," he says. "Reality sets in and you're going to do the things you have to do; you're not going to just abandon all responsibility. You're going to continue to deal with it. But—you're not going to let it cloud your life. I've got too many things I want to do. I've got too many things I'm doing now, so I don't think about it in that sense. I will take the necessary precautions that I must take—diet, exercise, have the testing on a regular basis. I can't say, 'No, I'm through with prostate cancer now' and never have another test. I don't think I could afford to do that."

Some of us aren't just thinking about the spread or return of our cancer; we're already living with it. Charlie is dealing with a growing tumor in his pelvic region. John's cancer has also metastasized. To date, there is no cure for systemic, metastasized prostate cancer, and that affects how those of us at this stage think, and the treatments we pursue.

*Lymph Node Metastasis.*   The lymph nodes are small bean-sized glands located throughout the body that filter lymphatic fluid. Lymphatic fluid from the prostate drains into several lymph nodes clustered on each side of the pelvis.

Lymph node metastasis is the spread of cancer to the lymph nodes via the lymph system. If cancer has spread to the lymph nodes, it has probably spread to other sites as well, most commonly to the bone, the bladder, and the bowel. Studies have shown that cancer spreads in 40–50 percent of men with positive lymph nodes in less than two years. In five years 75 percent of men develop distant metastases. Whether your cancer has spread to the lymph nodes is an important factor in deciding your course of treatment. Lymph node metastasis may cause a variety of symptoms including swellings you can feel in the pelvic area, pain due to urinary tract obstruction, and swelling in the lower limbs. (G. E. Hanks, Treatment of early stage prostate cancer: Radiotherapy. In V. T. DeVita Jr., S. Hellman, S. A. Rosenberg, eds. *Important Advances in Oncology.* Philadelphia: JB Lippincott, 1994:225–239; A. Yagoda, Genitourinary cancers. In J. S. MacDonald, D. G. Haller, R. J. Mayer, eds. *Manual of Oncologic Therapeutics,* 3rd ed. JB Lippincott, 1995:188–205.)

"I've been living with systemic cancer since 1991," Charlie said. "My decision to have a radical prostatectomy is always with me, every day, even though I feel and look very healthy."

"I've got cancer in my spine, my ribcage, and my arm," John told us. "I've had all the MRIs and the bone scans and continue to have them, but basically, I don't let it bother me. I'm looking at life, thankful for what has happened to date, based on the fact that I've seen some people in real pain with this disease. I'm talking about men with tears in their eyes. So far, that has not occurred to me. I take life on a day-to-day basis and see what happens."

"I'm refractory. I'm systemic, metastasized, and the tumor is growing," began Charlie.

"It's one-third larger than it was a year ago. My PSA is rising. But I am also an empowered patient," he continued. "I'm still fighting, reading, trying new things, and having serious talks with my three doctors and nutritionist. I will look everywhere for information and

## Research Update

The timing and choice of whether to treat confirmed or suspected recurrent prostate cancer after a radical prostatectomy is difficult and uncertain for both physician and patient. In patients who are suspected of having residual disease (positive margins, extracapsular disease, seminal vesicle or lymph node involvement), adjuvant therapy is often used. However, depending on the criteria used to determine the need for adjuvant treatment, 30–70 percent of patients may be exposed to the risks and costs of treatment unnecessarily—they may never have a recurrence. Conversely, if patients with local disease are left untreated, the cancer may have an opportunity to grow and spread before salvage treatment is started.

Currently, a persistent or subsequent elevation of PSA after a radical prostatectomy is the best method for the early detection of residual disease. The possibility that a therapeutic window exists between adjuvant therapy and therapy for a proven recurrence prompted researchers to evaluate the effectiveness of radiation in patients whose only evidence of disease after a radical prostatectomy is an elevated PSA level.

Forty-seven patients whose PSA was greater than 0ng/ml postoperatively had radiation to the pelvic area. After a median follow-up of 36 months, 64 percent of the patients had no evidence of disease (undetectable PSA), leading researchers to conclude that therapeutic radiation for these patients is highly effective.

Researchers also concluded that the optimal strategy after a prostatectomy is to observe patients regardless of pathological risk factors. If patients are found to have an elevated PSA (2ng/mg or less) and no overt metastatic disease on bone scans or CTs, a course of therapeutic radiation should be implemented. A PSA decrease during radiation confirms the presence of residual local disease.

Source: J. D. Forman, K. Meetze, E. Pontes, D. P. Wood, F. Shamsa, T. Rana, A. T. Porter. Therapeutic irradiation for patients with an elevated post-prostatectomy prostate specific antigen level. *Journal of Urology* 158 (1997):1436–1440.

seek every means to protect myself. I have a very healthy, up attitude, and I am going to do my best because I consider prostate cancer a challenge. I'm not afraid to die, and I'm going to push the envelope right to the end. With regards to treatment, I'm going to have a very open mind, but I am not going to focus on dying. I'm not go-

# Research Update

The progression of prostate cancer during androgen-deprivation therapy is a major clinical problem and the reasons it happens are poorly understood. Researchers are now looking at the androgen receptor (AR) gene for answers. Amplification of this gene was recently described in patients with recurrent prostate cancer who had not benefited from androgen-deprivation therapy.

To evaluate the hypothesis that amplification of this gene caused the therapy failure, researchers studied whether the amplified AR gene was structurally intact and whether tumors with AR amplification had distinct biological and clinical characteristics.

The data suggest that tumors that responded well to androgen deprivation are most likely to recur with AR amplification. Tumors that showed no response never contained AR amplification at the time of recurrence.

The results emphasize the close association between AR amplification and the failure of androgen-deprivation therapy. Data also substantiated the hypothesis that AR amplification is directly contributing to therapy failure by allowing cells to resume hormone-dependent growth.

Amplification occurs exclusively in the recurrent tumors from patients whose disease has progressed during the therapy. No amplified cells were found in the untreated primary tumors, many of which came from patients with late-stage metastatic prostate cancer. Thus, AR amplification is not involved in the genesis of prostate cancer; nor does it occur during the clinical progression of cancer in patients who have not received androgen-deprivation therapy.

The discovery of AR gene amplification and the emerging understanding of the molecular mechanisms of therapy failure may in the future translate into new therapy options for patients with prostate cancer. The results illustrate, contrary to popular belief, that recurrent hormone-refractory tumors may not always be androgen independent.

Source: P. Koivisto, J. Kononen, C. Palmberg, T. Tammela, E. Hyytinen, J. Isola, J. Trapman, K. Cleutjens, A. Noordzij, T. Visakorpi, O-P. Kallioniemi. Androgen receptor gene amplification: A possible molecular mechanism for androgen deprivation therapy failure in prostate cancer. *Cancer Research* 57 (1997): 314–319.

ing to be intimidated by anybody, the world, the impact of the environment, nothing, not even ideas. I'm going to live my life as fully and completely as I can."

"First of all, I think you have to be able to accept the fact that you have cancer to survive," added Peter. "You'll go crazy if you try and fight that fact. But I don't think that means that I'm not actively fighting it. In other words, acceptance does *not* mean, 'OK, cancer, do what you will with me.'"

"I've had failures with surgery, radiation, and the experimental drug Calcitrol," Peter continued. "Right now, I'm on combination hormonal therapy. But I know that won't last forever. I've never known anyone who's been on it successfully for 20 years. I've heard of 10 years. I've known someone at 5 years, but that's the extent of my knowledge of how long it might last. I don't know what I'll do when the CHT fails, but I am looking for that silver bullet—that still may come along." (See Chapter 4 for more information on hormonal therapy.)

As you've read, Bud was one of the first men in the United States to take combination hormonal therapy after it was approved by the FDA. "When my doctor told me that these new drugs might shrink my prostate and stop the growth of cancer, I had no qualms about it. It was approved in November of '89," he told us, "and I was fortunate enough to go on it in January 1990. I was also the first one to go on intermittent hormonal therapy in November of '90. [See Chapter 4 for more on intermittent hormonal therapy.] At the time, I remember asking the doctors, 'When can I go off this therapy?' and my doctors said, 'Nobody's ever gone off of it—nobody's ever tried.' I tried in 1990, and major cancer centers started trying this therapy in 1991. I'm fortunate that intermittent therapy has worked out favorably for me—so far."

"I think it was a commendable thing that you did," responded Paul. "When any new medicine comes out and you're one of the first ones to use it, you're at a higher risk than if you're using something that's been on the market for 30 years with a known history. If you're faced with that decision, you just have to be very careful, learn as much as you can about the new therapy, and weigh the pros and cons."

Like Bud, Don also decided to gamble and went off combination hormonal therapy after only a year. "I've been off CHT about two years and five months," Don told us. "Right now, I feel that continuing my alternative therapies is best for me. I'm on a hydrogen peroxide maintenance program that is 35 percent hydrogen peroxide in distilled water. I can 'soup' the amount of hydrogen peroxide up higher if I want, stay at that level, or come back down. It just depends on what my PSA does. Right now it's going up a little bit and is right around 3.5, but I still have a lot of alternatives. I'm taking lots of herbs. I can also go back on CHT, and if that fails, I could possibly go for the cryotherapy. But for the time being, I'm just going to wait a bit and see what happens."

"I think that one of the most important things we must do is to stay on a program of prevention," said Charlie, "and absolutely maintain a healthy body. That includes every one of us. Sometimes cancer patients who are fortunate to be in remission get lulled into a sense of false security. Don't! We are all in danger of a recurrence, and there are other major diseases involved, too, not just cancer. We must be alert to everything and stay on the program. That includes detoxifying and oxygenating our bodies as Don does. He is very much on a program and so am I. We all need to watch our diets to make sure we're getting the proper nutrients plus vitamins to smash those free radicals, and the proper supplements. That's not only good for us physically, but it's something positive on which to focus. In fact, it's good for the entire family. We need to keep track of our disease, keep track of our PSA, exercise daily, do whatever else is important to fight this disease. Stay on the program—regardless of the stage of your disease! That's a message I hope everyone who reads this book understands and follows."

Having a game plan is essential to all of us. That means staying abreast of the latest treatment options, and there are many. But you have to realize that this takes time and energy. And if you're wondering if you have the time to devote to this, all you have to do is ask yourself one question: "Is my life worth the time it takes to read this new article or listen to this discussion?" In fact, that's why most of us continue to attend support group meetings, search the Internet, and talk to other men with prostate cancer: Each entity is a tremendous source of information. And you never know what bit of new information you come across will make a difference.

As John pointed out, "Each time one of you fellows talk here at the retreat, I listen and I gain a little more knowledge, and to me that's the most important thing. When I go home, and I'm on the

---

## Research Update

One of the main goals in treating prostate cancer is androgen deprivation of the tumor. Many types of therapy have been evaluated including estrogen therapy, surgical castration, LHRH analogues, and antiandrogens, but there are limitations associated with each of these therapies.

For example, antiandrogens such as flutamide have a short half-life in the body. Concentrations decrease rapidly after a single dose and must be "supported" by additional daily doses. When patients don't comply with dosing, blood concentrations of the drug rapidly decrease, which allows any circulating androgen to restimulate tumor growth.

These limitations prompted a search for a drug that could be administered once daily to facilitate compliance and ensure efficacy and that would have better safety and tolerability profiles compared to flutamide and nilutamide.

Out of over 2,000 compounds specifically synthesized, the search yielded one successful candidate, the nonsteroidal antiandrogen bicalutamide (Casodex®). The antitumor activity of bicalutamide was demonstrated in cell models and in clinical studies and was observed to produce a more profound and complete androgen blockade than flutamide.

Bicalutamide, which has a longer half-life, is taken once a day and was well tolerated in the patients tested. The most frequently reported side effects were breast pain, gynecomastia, and hot flashes, but they rarely resulted in patients withdrawing from therapy.

Source: G.J.C.M. Kolvenbag, B.J.A. Furr. Bicalutamide ("Casodex") development: From theory to therapy. *Cancer Journal* 3, 4 (1997):192–203.

---

telephone to people who call from all across the country, I'm going to be able to provide them with even more information."

Peter put our time and involvement in perspective. "I would venture a guess that the average 'educational investment' by each of us here would easily exceed several hundred hours."

Are we worth it? Every second! It's called empowerment.

"I think that any future treatments for me will depend on where the 'beast' is when and if they find it," began Derek. "My PSA is still low, but it's rising steadily, which could be an indication that

---

## Treatments for Bone Pain

*Strontium-89 (Metastron®).*   Strontium-89 is a bone-seeking radioactive compound injected directly into the bloodstream and is used to treat bone pain for advanced cancer patients. After injection, Strontium-89 avoids healthy bone and is absorbed by the cancerous areas. This destroys prostate cancer cells, which reduces or eliminates pain. It takes about two weeks for Strontium-89 to achieve its full effect. If the pain returns, patients can have additional treatments. Strontium-89 can cause a drop in platelets, which are responsible for blood clotting, or in white blood cells, which are responsible for fighting against infection. Your platelet and white blood cell counts will be monitored during treatment.

*External-Beam Radiation.*   External-beam radiation is the focused delivery of radiation to a specific site to kill the cancer and to relieve symptoms such as bone pain. The treatment is aimed at the painful or problematic area and is given on an outpatient basis.

*Bisphosphonate.* Biophosphonates are drugs (etidronate, pamidronate ([Aredia®]), that block bone destruction. They are used in the treatment of hypercalcemia and to prevent bone fractures. They are also being used to treat bone pain.

*Samarium-153.*   Samarium-153 is a radioisotope being tested to relieve pain of bone metastases and other complications of advanced prostate cancer.

---

there's still some cancer left somewhere. I still have the option of having another cryotherapy procedure if the ultrasound and the biopsy show that the cancer is still confined to the capsule. If my PSA keeps rising as steadily as it has for the past two years, I'll probably first go back to Dr. Lee at Crittenton Hospital and have him take a look. If he can't find anything, then my best option is probably CHT, but only intermittently—and only after I get some more information and data on how best to do it."

"What will I do if my PSA starts to rise? I will probably go on CHT, too," Manuel told us. "I'm not sure, though. I'll have to make that decision when it comes. My doctor told me I had clear margins, but I know that is no guarantee. I know that it can still recur—two, three, five years down the line. And like I said, I'm preparing myself for it."

*Chemotherapy.* Chemotherapy is the use of chemicals to attack and kill cancer cells. The drugs circulate throughout the body and kill both cancer cells and rapidly dividing healthy cells, such as hair follicles, sperm, and blood cells. Standard chemotherapy, although it's an option, has not been proven to be highly effective in advanced prostate cancer, and there are side effects from the drugs to consider. However, depending on your circumstances, you and your doctor may decide that chemotherapy is the best treatment for you at the time—and it may help relieve disease symptoms such as pain. Dosages are continually being refined and, in addition, if you're taking a specific combination of drugs that fail, you may be able to try a different combination with better results. Currently, the FDA has approved only two drugs to treat hormone-resistant prostate cancer. They are estramustine (Emcyt®) and mitoxantrone (Novantrone®) plus glucocorticoid.

Prostate cancer can recur in the form of a tumor called small-cell carcinoma, especially in metastases to the liver and pelvis. Small-cell prostate cancers are similar to other small-cell cancers, such as lung, and may respond to the same kinds of chemotherapy drugs used to treat those tumors. A biopsy will tell you and your doctor what kind of tumor it is and what kind of chemotherapy may benefit you. (P. C. Walsh, J. G. Worthington. *The Prostate.* Baltimore, MD: Johns Hopkins University Press, 1995.)

Radiation therapy at this stage is also frequently used to relieve bone pain or to treat other symptoms. As with other treatments, your age, general health, and amount of disease and symptoms will help you decide on a specific treatment.

"I started on CHT when my bone scans showed some dark spots," said John, "but it only worked about ten months. Then they took me off flutamide and the PSA dropped, but then it suddenly started back up again. My oncologist is telling me to wait a little bit longer and see what happens. I still have the option of going on Casodex® which will probably bring my PSA down again, but I've never been able to get it down below 1. But you have to realize I still have my prostate. So we'll wait and see what happens. Right now I don't feel much pain. I do get a little twinge here and there. What I'm getting is a little hot poker feeling in my left leg between

## Research Update

Prostate cancer metastasizes most often to the pelvic lymph nodes and to the bone, with the most common symptom being pain. The role of chemotherapy in relieving symptoms of advanced disease (palliation) has been controversial, and many types of chemotherapy are poorly tolerated by patients.

A recent Canadian study investigated the benefit of chemotherapy in patients with symptomatic hormone-resistant prostate cancer. One hundred sixty-one patients were randomized to receive mitoxantrone plus prednisone or prednisone alone. Researchers chose pain relief as the primary indicator of palliation. The primary end point was a response defined as a 2-point decrease in pain as assessed by a 6-point pain scale completed by patients (or complete loss of pain if initially 1+).

Patients kept a diary in which they recorded all medications. A numeric scale was used to compute a daily analgesic score. Palliative response was observed in 23 of 80 patients who received mitoxantrone alone and in 10 of 81 patients who received prednisone alone. The duration of palliation was longer in patients who received chemotherapy. There was no difference in overall survival.

Treatment was well tolerated except for five episodes of possible cardiac toxicity in 130 patients who received mitoxantrone. Most responding patients had an improvement in quality-of-life scales and a decrease in PSA levels, leading researchers to conclude that chemotherapy with mitoxantrone and prednisone provides palliation for some patients with symptomatic hormone-resistant prostate cancer.

Source: I. F. Tannock, D. Osoba, M. R. Stockler, D. S. Ernst, A. J. Neville, M. J. Moore, G. R. Armitage, J. J. Wilson, P. M. Venner, C.M.L. Coppin, K. C. Murphy. Chemotherapy with mitoxantrone plus prednisone or prednisone alone for symptomatic hormone-resistant prostate cancer: A Canadian randomized trial with palliative end points. *Journal of Clinical Oncology* 15, 6 (1997):1756–1764.

my knee and my hip. The doctors think what's happening is that the buildup of calcium on the spine is starting to squeeze the spine and it's affecting some of those nerves in there. But I'm not ready for Strontium-89. I don't feel like I need that.

"I did get 13 additional radiation treatments last fall," John continued, "and like my previous experience, I had a problem swallowing from the radiation. But again, I was a guinea pig. In a sense,

# Research Update

Current chemotherapy has not been highly effective in the treatment of metastatic prostate cancer. Researchers say that the development of new therapeutic agents, preferably with novel mechanisms of action, is desirable.

Researchers in Germany report that the antitumor activity of the flavone flavopiridol has been selected for further studies based in part on its behavior in the anticancer drug-screening system of the National Cancer Institute. Flavonoids such as quercetin and genistein have been shown to inhibit tumor cell growth in vitro but are less potent than the new flavone flavopiridol and require higher concentrations for cytotoxic activity. Flavopiridol is synthesized from *Dysoxylum binectariferum,* a plant native to India.

Flavopiridol has been evaluated for antitumor activity in vitro and in vivo. In 23 human tumor models, flavopiridol was identified as a highly potent cytotoxic compound.

Eighteen human tumors established in nude mice and five cell-line-derived xenografts were used as tumor models for in vitro investigations. In vivo investigations were completed in nude mice bearing advanced-stage growing prostate cancer xenografts.

Antitumor activity in vitro of flavopiridol was observed even at very low concentrations of 0.1ng/ml in three of four prostatic xenografts and in one melanoma xenograft. Flavopiridol was considerably less potent when directed against human bone marrow. Toxicity in in vitro cultures was evident only at high concentrations of 100ng/ml, an important result indicating flavopiridol's potential for high selectivity for susceptible prostate tumor cells.

Researchers concluded that flavopiridol showed strong prostate antitumor activity in vitro. The prostate antitumor activity is also reflected by the in vivo models studied. Initial clinical efforts with flavopiridol might consider early evaluation in patients with prostate cancer. Further studies are necessary to outline the action of flavopiridol in concert with conventional chemotherapeutic agents.

Source: M. Drees, W. A. Dengler, T. Roth, H. Labonte, J. Mayo, L. Malspeis, M. Grever, E. A. Sausville, H. H. Fiebig. Flavopiridol (L86–8275): Selective antitumor activity *in vitro* and activity *in vivo* for prostate carcinoma cells. *Clinical Cancer Research* 3 (1997):273–279.

## New or Unique Therapies

*Ketoconazole (Nizoral®).*   Ketoconazole is an FDA-approved anti-fungal agent that can be effective in prostate cancer by blocking the production of testosterone from the testicles and androgens made by the adrenal glands. However, ketoconazole can suppress the production of steroids produced in the adrenal glands and should be prescribed with a corticosteroid such as prednisone. (Not yet FDA approved for the treatment of prostate cancer.)

*Paclitaxel (Taxol®).*   Paclitaxel is a natural product of the plant *Taxus brevifolia* that appears to hold promise for useful activity in hormone-refractory prostate cancer. This use of paclitaxel is currently in clinical studies.

*Nilutamide (Nilandron®).*   Nilutamide is an FDA-approved antiandrogen used in combination hormonal therapy or in combination with an orchiectomy.

we're all guinea pigs because we all react differently to this disease and to the therapies.

"As far as chemotherapy goes, I won't take any. I've had four friends who had chemo last year. All four are dead. So I figure the batting average isn't that great. And my oncologist knows what my feelings are about this."

"The problem with chemotherapy," said Paul, "is that we don't have chemotherapy, yet, that works well. Prostate cancer is just different from other types of cancer."

"One thing I find in our support group," said John, "is that any little new thing that we hear raises hope. And you have to look at this from a positive standpoint and say, 'Well, this is wonderful.' But oftentimes there's a rise in hope—and then a fall. You're on a high—then suddenly you're on a low. It's hard sometimes."

"It's very hard," said Paul. "But I've got a lot of hope. I had an orchiectomy, cryotherapy, and am taking flutamide. I feel that I've beaten this cancer so far back that I can seriously think about the possibility of testosterone shots in the future. And there are always new therapies coming out."

Your fight against cancer gets even more complicated because doctors' opinions on what therapy or treatment you should use will vary tremendously. For example, there's ongoing controversy on whether to use antiandrogens and which antiandrogen works best. Should you try chemotherapy or watch and wait instead? That will depend on you, your individual case, and your doctor. Which brings us back to the point we made earlier: Every case of prostate cancer is different. And every patient reacts differently to the different therapies.

In addition, physicians have to be aware of any other medical problems that may exist in each of their patients. Since prostate cancer generally occurs in older men, there may be heart disease, diabetes, or other conditions to deal with in conjunction with prostate cancer. So what works for one man may not work for another and vice versa. You have to find the treatment plan that works for you, and the only way you'll be able to do that is to stay informed, work closely with your doctor—and keep trying.

According to Charlie, the treatment of cancer is like a pyramid. "When you're first diagnosed, you've got a pretty broad base of information and lots of options. It's stable stuff and the risks are well defined. A lot of people have probably had the treatment you're considering. When you're at that basic level, that large base of the pyramid, you're on the ground, and you know what's happening. If you don't get a good result from that, then you climb up the pyramid a little more. Now you're a little higher off the ground, and your options are beginning to narrow because you're at a different level. And you may be facing a newly approved drug where there isn't quite as much experience, quite as many success data to go on. Then we get to clinical trials and the new experimental therapies that are pushing you to higher levels on the pyramid. And as you go up the pyramid, because nothing is working, there are more risks and more uncertainties because your condition is getting worse. You have fewer options, and finally, you get to the top. You get to the point that you either jump off the pyramid or just sit there. But you can't sit there forever because you're not going to last. So you can take a risk on this newest clinical trial and see if it works for you.

"I think clinical trials are choices," continued Charlie. "They're options that depend on you and your condition. Whether you take that choice or not depends, partly, on how successful you've been with previous treatments. It's kind of like looking at a chessboard and seeing that you've got a certain number of moves left to try and win the game."

Participation also depends on a number of other factors. It depends on your doctor's knowledge of studies, whether an appropri-

*Clinical Studies.*   Clinical studies are organized research programs that try to improve on standard treatments or answer specific questions about new treatments. For many patients, clinical studies offer hope after standard treatments have failed. Some patients may choose a clinical study well before treatment failure because they and their doctors feel this may be the best option. These studies may involve drug therapies, equipment or devices, or quality-of-life measures such as diet or exercise. All clinical studies for these new drugs or devices are monitored closely throughout by the sponsor and the FDA. In prostate cancer, there are several new drug therapies currently being tested, as well as methods of drug delivery.

All drug studies compare a new product or regimen with a proven product or regimen that is usually thought to be state-of-the-art. There is a randomized placement of patients into either the test group or the standard-of-care group. Although you may or may not benefit personally, your participation may affect the future of cancer care and may also help other cancer patients. Thus you'll want to carefully weigh the risks and benefits with your loved ones and your health care team before you make your decision.

Things to think about:

- What is the purpose of the study?
- Do I meet the requirements for participating in the study?
- What kinds of tests and treatments are involved?
- Do I have the time and energy to commit to the study? How could it affect my daily life?
- Will the timing of the treatments, tests, and clinic visits fit into my schedule? How long will the study last?
- Will I have to be hospitalized?
- Are the treatment choices safe for me? What are the potential side effects?
- If I am harmed as a result of the research, what treatment would I receive?

*(continues)*

ate study is available for you, whether you fit all the precise criteria for that study, and what your other options are. All these factors will play a role in your decision.

"If my stage of cancer had been determined to be in its final stages," said Bob, "and I knew that there was no other hope, I would agree to clinical trials at a time like that. But I don't think I

*(continued)*

- What are my other choices for treatment and how do the advantages and disadvantages compare?
- Do some participants in the study receive a placebo, or no treatment? If so, does the study have a "crossover" phase where the placebo group, or no-treatment group, will get the study treatment?
- What happens if I don't respond to the treatment?
- What are the potential benefits to me of participating in the study?
- What happens if I decide to quit during the study?
- When will I know the results?
- Will I have any expenses?
- What type of long-term follow-up care is part of the study?

All patients in the United States who are offered participation in a clinical study must, by law, receive informed-consent material to review and a copy of any signed document to take home. These materials and forms describe the purpose, benefits, risks, and procedures of the research study. If you decide that clinical trials are not for you, you may be able to receive an investigational drug in a compassionate-use program instead.

For specific NCI site locations of prostate cancer studies call the National Cancer Institute at 1–800–4–Cancer or log onto the NCI website at http://cancernet.nci.nih.gov. There are also privately funded corporate studies. Check with individual pharmaceutical companies for corporate studies.

For general information about clinical trials ask for the booklet *What Are Clinical Trials All About?* NCI, 1992 (available in English or Spanish).

For more information: Clinical trials in relapsed prostate cancer: Defining the target. *Journal of the National Cancer Institute* 88, 22 (Nov. 20, 1996).

would want to step out on that limb knowing that it might not work—that I could do more damage to myself than I would have if I hadn't volunteered for the clinical trial. But if I were in my last stages, and I knew there was nothing else—I've tried everything and I'm not getting any better and death is imminent—then I would say, 'Well if you need me, take me!'"

*Gene Therapy.*   Gene therapy involves the transfer of new genetic material into the cancer cells of a patient. Scientists have recently found the approximate location of a mutant gene that can increase the risk of prostate cancer. Carriers of this gene, called HPC-1 (hereditary prostate cancer–1), have almost a 90 percent chance of developing prostate cancer by age 85 compared to about a 20 percent lifetime risk for the general population. Researchers are hoping to find the defective gene and ultimately develop a test to determine who carries it. A metastasis suppresser gene has also been identified in rat prostate cancer cells. Further studies are planned to analyze the functions of this gene and evaluate the role it plays.

Researchers are also focusing on how gene therapy might help men with prostate cancer. Genetic discoveries may also have other long-range benefits. New findings may lead to better treatment of prostate cancer with existing therapies depending on tumor genetics. (*Journal of the National Cancer Institute* 88, 14 [August 17, 1996].)

There are many other variations of gene therapy under investigation and development. Most of these studies are in very early stages. As such, they involve a small number of patients and the requirements to qualify are very restrictive.

*Tumor Vaccines.*   Tumor vaccines are a type of immunotherapy being developed to prevent recurrences of the cancer or to get the body to reject the cancer. Some studies are looking at ways to deliver hormone-gene combinations to cancerous cells, which will trick the cancer cell into shuting down. Tumor vaccine studies also exploit the ability of cytokines to increase antitumor activity. Cytokines are naturally occurring substances in the body that help promote antitumor activity and help boost your natural immunity. Cancer cells are taken from the tumor, cultured, and enhanced with cytokine genes. These cells are reintroduced into the patient to stimulate immune response against cancer cells by natural killer cells. Studies in animals have shown long-lasting antitumor immunity.

For more information: *Understanding Gene Testing,* NCI/NIH Publication No. 96–3905, December 1995. Call 1–800–4-CANCER to order.

"I feel like Bob does," said Peter. "If I'd run the route and there was nothing I hadn't tried and the doctors were saying, 'Sorry' but there was a clinical trial that hopefully was going to address my stage of the problem, then I would probably elect to go on it. In fact, that came up much earlier when my surgery and radiation failed. At that time, my oncologist discussed with me the possibility of going into an NCI trial right then and there. We went ahead and applied for it, but as it turned out, I wasn't eligible. Patients had to be hormone refractory, and at that point I wasn't. And I'm glad it didn't happen. So I've been there on the threshold, and I wouldn't go there again unless I'd gotten to the point of feeling that I'd exhausted all other options."

"I think clinical trials definitely have a place," said Manuel. "Somebody has to do it. When I was in elementary school, I learned about an heroic act, back in Cuba at the turn of the century, that forever changed the course of living conditions in tropical areas. Dr. Carlos Findlay and Dr. Walter Reed advanced a theory that mosquitoes caused yellow fever. A group of Carmelite priests offered themselves for experimentation to see if it was true. They gave their lives. They died because they were inoculated with an extract of mosquitoes, and their sacrifice proved that the mosquito was the culprit who transmitted the disease. So there is a place for clinical trials, and in many ways, that would be the giving of yourself for a very good cause. If I got to that point, I wouldn't take it lightly, but I wouldn't mind participating if I felt I had the call to do that."

"There's also another aspect of this," said Paul. "Not all clinical studies are 'I'm dying, this is my last breath' type of thing. For example, there are ongoing studies of drugs to determine if they will act as a preventative of prostate cancer. There were certain qualifications. For example, you had to be over 55, and some of the guys were getting placebos and some were getting the real thing."

"In a sense I'm on a clinical trial," John told us, "but it's the Chinese herbs. I'm still taking my other pills. I still have that treatment base, so I'm not giving up anything. I'm just seeing if the herbs help, and it's only a 45-day trial period. I have a PSA this week. Then, when I finish the herbs, I'll have another PSA. I can continue doing that, but if I don't have positive results, I'll just quit and go back on the Essiac tea and some of the other things I was doing before. I believe that decisions are made day to day, and you make one when new information is put before you. If I were eligible for a clinical trial that involved some new medicine and I had to give up some of my current medication and I didn't know which direction the new medicine could go, I would not go on it. I'd really want to check into it to see if I wanted to do this before I said yes. To me, I can see

> ### *Provisions for Death*
>
> #### by Cindy Stults (Peter's wife)
>
> *Today my husband*
> *signed a will*
> *leaving his 1988 Cherokee Jeep,*
> *equity in our home,*
> *stock in our business,*
> *and a cardboard box filled with*
> *forty years of Kodak pictures*
> *to me.*
> *There is no mention*
> *of who will share*
> *my coffee*
> *in the morning.*

progress, but I'm not going to be a guinea pig to the point where I'm going to stop my other medication."

It all comes down to personal choice and quality of life.

## End-of-Life Issues

As Paul says, "We're all going to die sooner or later, but I'm going to procrastinate as much as possible." No one ever likes to think about dying. "But with the diagnosis of any disease," says Peter, "comes a reminder of our own personal fragileness and vulnerability." In fact, you can't help thinking about it.

"The thought of dying young, at 65 or even 75, never occurred to me until I had this diagnosis," Peter remembers. "In my family, everyone always lives 'forever.' My father died this year at 96. My mom is 91 and is still going strong. So I never gave death a second thought. Now, I've learned to accept my mortality. I recognize it, but I'm more concerned for my wife and child in some ways than I am for myself. I have a 14-year-old son, so I'm particularly bothered more than anything else by the thought of not being here when he graduates from high school or college."

Death is a topic that's difficult enough to think about by yourself. It can be an even tougher topic to broach with loved ones. Peter has

*Will.*   A will is an important legal document that spells out how you want your property distributed when you die, with a minimum delay. You can name a trusted family member, friend, or professional to handle your personal affairs, known as an executor. It is preferable to seek the advice of a lawyer so that decisions about taxes, beneficiaries, and asset distribution will be legally binding.

*Trust.*   A trust is an arrangement under which one person or institution, called the trustee, holds the title to property for the benefit of other persons called beneficiaries. Trusts can be used to defer estate taxes until the death of the second spouse. Trusts are especially useful for lifetime management of large estates where there is a substantial amount of property and professional management is desired. They have a high level of acceptance in the business and financial community.

Things to think about when setting up a trust:

- Professionally managed trusts can be costly to set up and manage.
- A trust can create problems for public benefit eligibility (i.e., if you wish the public to benefit in any way from your estate).
- A trust can be set up as a "standby" to be used only in the case of incapacity.
- Use of a trust may have important tax consequences.

found that talking to his son gradually and in stages has helped both of them.

"When I was first diagnosed, I just talked to my youngest child, who was nine at the time, about my having a diseased organ that needed to be removed. I don't think my wife and I even mentioned cancer. And then when it recurred, we identified it as being cancer and what the treatments were at that time. At each stage and advancement of the cancer we've talked more with him, but I've tried not to focus on it—to frighten him. He's very aware that I have prostate cancer and he's very aware that it's a dangerous disease. Of course, he hears me talking to all sorts of people who call me just after they've been diagnosed. We get into extensive discussions on the phone, and I know he's overheard a lot of that. As time goes on and he grows older—and I survive—I'll certainly be talking to him more about it.

"I haven't talked a great deal about death to my wife," Peter continued. "Illness and death happen to frighten my wife. But even before the cancer, when we talked about estate planning and started to talk about life insurance, she really couldn't do it. That's a very difficult subject for her, so there hasn't been a lot of discussion—and I don't force it. I keep touching on it but only go as far as she's able."

"On the legal side of everything," said Paul, "I took a more serious interest in trying to be prepared after I was diagnosed. I don't have much, but what little I have I tried to put into a form that would be easier for my wife and children to access and take advantage of and not lose half of it. I contrast this with getting run over, in an accident or something. I've had the time to take care of financial arrangements and do some things I've wanted to do. I've also made the funeral arrangements."

The funeral arrangements may be made, but Phyllis doesn't think they'll be needed any time soon. "Sometimes, to hear him tell it, the situation sounds pretty bad. And I don't know if all men are this way, but it seems that they all have the feeling that we women are going to outlive them, and we're going to be around much longer than they are. And I keep telling him, 'I hate to disappoint you, but someday I may just drop dead, and you're going to have to figure all this out for yourself.' I think in some ways he's probably healthier than I am. But I expect our future to be long and happy."

"Both Manuel and I have living wills," said Mary, "because we went through hell when my mother died. She was seriously ill, and had a 'do not resuscitate' (DNR) on her hospital charts—and when her heart failed, they revived her anyway. So that opened a whole series of problems, as she lingered and suffered unnecessarily, and we did not want our children to have to go through the hell that we went through. Manuel also has a legal will that he had drawn up before he had his surgery. I don't have mine completed yet, but I have a handwritten will. We did this because we have his children and mine, so it was very important to us to clearly state how to dispose of our bodies. Our wishes are to be cremated. We both know this, and we've talked about it. Manuel is sure he's going to die before me, but you never know."

"Men always assume that they're going to go first," observed Rosalie. "There are some very surprised men in our neighborhood

*Advance Directive.* An advance directive is a legal document that allows you to convey your decisions about your health care before you become too ill to make them. You must make these wishes known to your physician and loved ones so that they will carry out your wishes if you become disabled or unable to communicate with them.

*Living Will.* A living will is a legal document stating your wishes about life-sustaining medical care and conditions under which you want to be kept alive or allowed to die. It is used if you become terminally ill, incapacitated, or unable to communicate. Everyone has the right to accept or refuse medical care. A living will protects your rights and removes the decisionmaking burden from family and friends.

Remember: Your decision to not receive "aggressive medical treatment" is not the same as withholding all medical care. When your goal of treatment becomes comfort and maintaining your quality of life, you can still request antibiotics, nutrition and fluids, pain medication, radiation therapy, and other interventions.

whose wives had the nerve to go and die on them. It threw all their financial planning off."

Bob's choice of profession mandated preplanning and precipitated peace of mind. "I made my funeral arrangements about 20, 25 years ago," said Bob. "This is a subject that's talked about when you come out of the Police Academy. As you're getting ready to leave there, they talk about the possibility that your life is on the line, and it behooves you to have your business in order so that there won't be a lot of legal tangles to deal with later on. So I made mine early on, and I've talked about death quite a bit throughout my life, so it's kind of like a normal conversation thing. When it's going to happen, it's going to happen, so you just deal with it. For me, having that kind of attitude is kind of a "freeing" thing. And the arrangements were made way before I had prostate cancer. I've chosen to be cremated—so there won't be much dealing with the old body. It's going to go up in smoke."

"I've also chosen to be cremated," said Peter. "My family owned an island off the west coast of Florida. We sold the island, but we still consider it ours. When Dad died this year, he was cremated, and the whole family went down there, including some grandkids, and

> *Durable Power of Attorney.*   A durable power of attorney is a legal
> document through which one person (the principal) gives legal au-
> thority to another (the agent) to act on his or her behalf. With a
> legal power of attorney, you are basically appointing someone to
> manage any part or all of your financial or personal affairs. You
> can include instructions, guidelines, or limitations as you wish.
> Most states require that the document be signed and notarized.
>
> *Medical Power of Attorney.*   A medical power of attorney is the
> same as a durable power of attorney but directed exclusively at
> health care concerns. It lets you appoint another person to make
> any or all health care decisions for you and to spell out guidelines
> for those decisions if you become incapacitated. Creating this doc-
> ument usually requires the same legal arrangements as a durable
> power of attorney, but special statutory requirements exist in
> some states.

we went around the island in a little boat, slowly scattering his
ashes all the way around his island. That's what I want to do, too. I
want to have my ashes scattered around the island where my Dad's
are."

"Don's nephew knows the creek and the rocks where Don's ashes
are supposed to go," began Lynne.

Don continued, "My favorite hunting spot is in the Upper Penin-
sula of Michigan—way up where they have 300 inches of snow on
these high mountain tops—and my ashes are going to go a little bit
here, a little bit there.

"I've still got tremendous hope that I'll beat this thing, though.
When I was 18 years old, I went to my army physical and I turned
up 4-F. The doctors told me I was going to die in six months. I had
blood in my urine, and they told me I had a prostate of an 80-year-
old when I was 18. Anyway, I haven't died yet, so again, I'm still
hoping. And the thought of dying doesn't really bother me too much
because I have a good wife who's going to carry on and take care of
the family."

"Does she shoe horses, too?" asked Virgil.

"No, she doesn't have to do that," smiled Don. "She's got her
own business going."

"And I'm fine with all this early preparation," said Lynne. "We've
also been very open with all our kids. They all understand. Don

even jokes about it with them. As far as having a living will—one of the reasons we haven't spent a lot of time on this is we had a bad experience with them. I took care of an elderly woman for 13 years, and we tried to set up everything like that ahead of time so everything would go smoothly. But in our case none of it worked. Part of the reason for all the hassles we had were that the laws in Michigan are constantly changing. So one piece of advice is, know what's happening in your state."

"One of the results of my diagnosis," Peter told us, "is that I felt I had an obligation to get my affairs in order. I basically left the business world in order to protect the business that I owned. I resigned as president and made my wife president. So far, it's worked out quite well. I miss the business, but I felt that was something I had to do. I also went to my lawyer and redid my wills. I remember that I spent a tremendous amount of time on those things that first year after diagnosis. It was something I could do and I think it was a matter of not knowing what else to do. I felt a responsibility to my family, and I had a need to do *something*. As I look back, I think that's the reason I spent so much time on it. Then I started learning more about the disease, feeling more in control, and to be honest, I haven't looked at the will in the last five years."

"Never once did I think I wasn't going to make it," Bud remembered, "but what I was really shooting for was to have five years to get my estate and everything in line and maybe change a few things. I didn't have to change too much because I had everything pretty well under control, but I still felt the need to take a close look at the legal end of things. Now I'm seven years out from my diagnosis!"

"Mostly I'm just trying to spend my kids' inheritance," joked Derek. "My significant other and I are having a hell of a good time right now enjoying life, and I haven't made a whole lot of arrangements about how my assets will be spread out. I had a living will, but that needs to be updated and changed a little. I just haven't done it—yet."

"In terms of mortality, it depends on the seriousness of the disease," said Charlie. "If you're facing this disease with no options, you're going to be a lot more concerned. And if you're in the very early stages or you had an apparently 'successful' radical prostatectomy or cryotherapy or whatever and you're a survivor, then you're not going to focus on it too much. But when you really think you're still a patient, like me, and you are sick and it's kind of serious, then

*Hospice.* If you are dealing with end-of-life issues, hospice care is a program that can help you manage your symptoms, control your pain, and provide emotional support to you and your family. Besides a nurse, who will make regularly scheduled visits to your home, a hospice team usually includes a social worker, home health aides, a chaplain, and volunteers. It's a team of experts whose job is to help your family and provide skilled care to you—so you can remain in your home. Sometimes your hospice team can help arrange for needed medical equipment such as canes, walkers, wheelchairs, or special beds. Some hospices also have facilities where people can stay if care at home becomes impossible. In many of these facilities, the patient is allowed to bring personal possessions such as photos, pictures for the walls, rugs, chairs, and other possessions to make the surroundings comfortable and familiar. Some even allow pets.

In most cases, to be eligible for a hospice program, you must be diagnosed as having less than six months to live. Most hospices require that you are no longer receiving "curative" therapy. However, therapy that helps to control disease symptoms such as irradiation to metastases sites or chemotherapy that may relieve pain may be allowed. The goal is symptom management and quality of life until death occurs.

Because symptom management is so important to your quality of life, most hospice programs advise that you enter a program as soon as you are eligible—instead of waiting until the last few weeks or days of life. The cost of hospice care varies depending on the services provided. Hospice care is covered under most private insurance plans, Medicare, and Medicaid. For a local referral or to learn more about hospice care, call

- your local Visiting Nurse Association (VNA),
- your health care provider or local hospital,
- the Hospice Education Institute (1–800–331–1620),
- the National Hospice Organization (1–800–658–8898).

your view of it changes. The religious part of it I've settled pretty well in my own mind—the Bible promises resurrection. The burial part is settled, too. My parents are buried at Notre Dame, and I found out that I also could be buried at Notre Dame—and that's a big deal. In our family, that is a huge part of our culture for lots of reasons. That added just another whole 'happy' dimension to the whole thing, which made it easier for me to think about it. So now, I know that eventually I will die—when or why, I don't know. I am not afraid of it, at least that's what I say today. Whether I will change that position, we'll just have to see."

"The big frustration for me is that there's no cure," began John. "I always think in terms of if something went wrong, I could fix it. But here's something that can't be fixed. I know I don't want to be a guinea pig to some of these doctors. And I don't want chemo or radiation because I had so many problems with radiation. So what the heck—if I die two months sooner, it isn't going to make any difference to me. We've got wills. We change them as they're required to be changed, and we already have our cemetery plots. We don't have any children to take care of. For some reason I feel I'm here until a certain time. When the Man calls, I'm going to go."

"I guess," said Rosalie, "that since we've become active in US TOO, we've been to so many memorial services and funerals that we realize more and more that the quality of life is very important. And I hate to say it, but a lot of the doctors are using patients as guinea pigs. They're putting people through horrendous stuff, and they don't have a clue! They just want to use their bodies."

"The frustrating thing," continued John, "is that somebody calls up and says, 'I've got a PSA of 2,000 or 4,000.' Well, what do you say to a person like that? We've had people with PSAs of three and four, and the doctor says, 'Get your things in order. You're only going to live six months.' Those are the guys you want to talk to because that's what you're there for—to reassure them that, hey, the end of the world hasn't come. I was diagnosed with prostate cancer five years ago. How long the cancer had been growing prior to that, I don't know. But we take life day to day. Rosalie's involved in many things, so if I die ahead of her, she'll be able to continue on. Life goes on."

"We have come to the conclusion," said Rosalie, "that quality of life is more important than length of life. We've already rejected things that the doctors wanted to do. We felt it would be more negative than positive. We already know about hospice care and we're not really happy with the way some of the hospices are run. Certainly not all of them, but some sort of warehouse these people, and in some cases we've seen some people do better at home with people who will take a more personal interest in them.

"What would I do if John was dying? I would keep him at home as long as I possibly could. I would hire whatever help I had to keep

Some books you may find helpful:

*Anatomy of the Spirit: The Seven Stages of Power and Healing.* Caroline Myss, Ph.D. New York: Three Rivers Press (a division of Crown Publishers), 1996.

*Why People Don't Heal and How They Can.* Carolyn Myss, Ph.D. New York: Harmony Books (a division of Crown Publishers), 1997.

*A Year to Live, How to Live This Year as if It Were Your Last.* Stephen Levine. New York: Harmony Books (a division of Crown Publishers), 1997.

him comfortable and feeling at ease. However, we put our emphasis not on thinking about funerals and death but on living life one moment, one hour, one day at a time. We're not ignoring this. We've been through many, many of these ceremonies and we have a whole liturgy in our church, so he and I know what to expect.

"But I really believe that we're here to celebrate life. Not to dwell on death. If you really have this idea that your life is an ending but that your soul is immortal, then this is just a rite of passage all of us are going through."

In fact, our closing thoughts for this chapter can be summed up in two words: optimism and hope.

"I've always been an optimist," said Peter, "but since the disease, other than the times I've fallen into a deep pit of despair, as we all have, I'm probably more optimistic, have a more optimistic view of the whole world—of myself, my family, and my friends—in part because I think it's essential. It's essential to my overall health and to my fight against cancer."

"The key here," concluded John, "is that I'm not going to sit down, look at the wall, and say, 'What have you done to me, God? Why me?' Why *not* me? I'm encouraged. I'm optimistic that in time a solution will be found. But am I worried about it? I'm concerned about it, but I'm not worried about it yet. Because there's nothing I can do except try and keep ahead of this disease—and keep hope alive."

# 1 0

# *Advocacy and Education*

## TOWARD A CURE

*That's why I always tell people to have faith and hope, because we're so close. We just may come over the line and conquer this thing.*

—*Bud Irish*

After "listening" to our conversations thus far, you probably won't be surprised that the subject matter of this chapter has nearly captured our souls. We are advocates; advocates for the 44,000 men who will die from this disease every year, for the men and their families who are living with prostate cancer today, and for the more than 209,000 men who will be newly diagnosed each year.

What do we want? It's quite simple, really. We want more awareness about prostate cancer so that men will be screened and diagnosed earlier. We want every man to have a compassionate and open-minded doctor at the time of diagnosis and through the course of his treatment. We want every man armed with the information he needs to make informed decisions. We want better, more effective treatments. We want a cure. That will take time, energy, commitment—and money.

Charlie told us that he'd been waiting for this discussion ever since the retreat began. Without mincing words, he began. "I've listened to breast cancer advocates describe what their organizations have done in terms of finance, organization, structure, political clout—everything you have to do to be successful. If you benchmark the condition of the prostate cancer activist groups, compared to breast cancer and AIDS, we are at the Cro-Magnon level!

---

## Research Update

In January 1997, the American Cancer Society estimated that 334,500 new cases of prostate cancer might occur in the United States during 1997. That projection was largely influenced by the rapid increase in incidence rates of prostate cancer during the late 1980s and early 1990s, probably related to the effects of the widespread use of PSA screening. The incidence rates also included a sharp decline between 1992 and 1993.

Incidence rates of prostate cancer for the years 1994 and 1995 also declined, but these rates were not available when the original estimates were made. Based on the new information, the ACS and the NCI concluded that the original 1997 projection was too high. The revised estimate of new prostate cancer cases is now approximately 209,900.

It is not known whether the incidence rate of prostate cancer will decline to the level seen before the initiation of PSA screening or approach a different level related to real changes in incidence.

Source: P. A. Wingo, S. Landis, L. A. G. Ries. An adjustment to the 1997 estimate for new prostate cancer cases. *CA: A Cancer Journal for Clinicians* 47 (1997): 239–242.

---

"Number one, we don't have a lot of people who are diagnosed with this disease who become activists. Number two, we're lousy at raising money, and thirdly, we have almost no political clout. The breast cancer group went out and knocked the doors down. These women were unreal. They pounded on doors. They gave money. They got fired from their jobs. They never gave up at building an organization as if they were building a business. And they never gave up trying to raise money. They used their relationships and their contacts to get on television and used the big names on TV to raise the consciousness of breast cancer. They talked to women's groups. They did a whole, giant, unrelenting, unselfish long-term campaign of the hardest work you could ever believe, and that's how they succeeded."

"One of the things that has propelled the AIDS movement is that it has become mainstream," said Virgil. "You had Elizabeth Taylor and all of Hollywood getting behind it. You had everyone in the New York garment industry getting behind it. In the breast cancer area you had every major magazine promoting the awareness of breast cancer and any number of corporate executives getting behind it. I want to do the same thing for prostate cancer. I want to go after a Forbes type to be able to get these guys who are in that same peer group, who control vast resources, to get them on the bandwagon. They are in the age group where they're at risk, so they've got more of an incentive and imperative to be there."

"We can see by the statistics that in regards to money, breast cancer and AIDS are way beyond us," said Paul. "But you have to keep in mind that the AIDS activists are for the most part younger men that are very viable and active in doing this sort of thing. I've been to prostate cancer support groups where it's clear that a lot of the people get prostate cancer later on in life and their interests are oftentimes laissez-faire—'let me die peacefully'—not everyone, but a lot of the men. In our group, we have some people who come and attend just one meeting, and we never see them again. We have just a small percentage who come to every meeting."

To be fair, not everyone is comfortable attending support groups, and not everyone wants to be an advocate for change—or has the energy. However, the cause needs bodies, and the more individuals who can join us, the better.

"Right now, I'm very much encouraged," said John, "especially because of all that's happened in the last six to eight months. Prostate cancer is starting to have a lot of publicity. We're getting articles in *Fortune Magazine* and *Time*. We're getting discussions on the talk shows, and this is very important for all of us."

Why is publicity and political influence important? Prostate cancer must be recognized by Congress and the general public as a major health concern for men, their families, and society. Without elevated awareness and a demonstrated need, federal and private research money will continue to bypass this disease in favor of more visible, more vocal, and more politically powerful ones.

For example, if you compare federal research funding for prostate cancer, breast cancer, and AIDS, you'll find some glaring discrepancies. The discrepancies are even greater when you further compare death rates and incidence rates. In 1996, AIDS topped the list with $1.62 billion; breast cancer followed with $550 million, and prostate cancer was at $80 million—barely a blip on the screen.

But our goal is not to fuel the funding wars between the sexes or between diseases. We are not at odds with the women and men with breast cancer or AIDS. We are also well aware that cancer research

## Research Update

Despite considerable scientific effort, relatively little is known about the biological events that cause the initiation and progression of prostate cancer. The development of new strategies for the treatment of prostate cancer demands an increased understanding of the cellular and molecular events involved in how prostate cancer starts and metastasizes.

Rodent models have provided valuable insights into the biology and pathology of primary prostate cancer and for assessing treatment strategies. But difficulty in establishing long-term human prostate epithelial cell lines has impeded efforts to understand how prostate cancer starts and to develop alternative therapies for the disease.

In a recent study, researchers successfully generated 14 immortal benign or malignant human tumor cell lines derived from primary adenocarcinomas of the prostate. Tissue specimens were obtained from six patients undergoing radical prostatectomies. Tissues designated as normal prostate, prostate cancer, or normal seminal vesicle were dissected separately for the purpose of generating cell cultures. The cell cultures have been successfully generated for more than one year.

Researchers say that such stable and long-term cultures are mandatory for biological, genetic, and immunological studies that will accelerate the development of new forms of prevention and therapy for the disease.

Source: R. K. Bright, C. D. Vocke, M. R. Emmert-Buck, P. H. Duray, D. Solomon, P. Fetsch, J. S. Rhim, W. M. Linehan, S. L. Topalian. Generation and genetic characterization of immortal human prostate epithelial cell lines derived from primary cancer specimens. *Cancer Research* 57 (1997):995–1002.

often overlaps, and as Paul pointed out, discoveries in one cancer can often end up benefiting another.

"I don't know a whole lot about how medicines get developed," observed Paul, "but it seems to me if researchers just focus on breast cancer, for example, maybe we're cutting ourselves off from all the other benefits of things. Sometimes researchers find that a particular medicine didn't really work on what they were originally aiming at, but it did work for some other problem."

A good example of this is the drug estramustine. It was originally targeted to breast cancer but was found to work better in advanced prostate cancer. (Estratmustine combined with the drug taxotere is also showing some good results.) Goserelin, another drug for advanced prostate cancer, was recently approved for use in advanced breast cancer.

That's not to say that more prostate cancer-specific research isn't desperately needed. It definitely is. The lack of federal money allocated to this disease is a slap in the face to the thousands of men battling this disease. But according to some leading researchers at the National Cancer Institute (NCI), there are also nonfinancial roadblocks that are preventing necessary research from getting done. Specifically, it's been difficult to get men to enter clinical studies, slowing the progress of critical research. Advocacy groups on the breast cancer side, however, have been very successful in getting women to sign up.*

However, money—or the lack thereof—continues to be the highest hurdle. Make no mistake, we *are* advocating that more money be spent on prostate cancer, but we are not saying less should be spent on other cancers. One solution lies in lobbying for increased funding for all medical research—which will benefit everyone. In other words, let's level the playing field.

"But first, we've got to push for more awareness, and we need all the help we can get," said Virgil. "You've got to make it personal. If, all of a sudden, you get your child to say, 'Daddy, I don't want you to die,' that to me is going to force the issue of awareness."

"I think that all we need is just a little break," said John, "and everyone is going to jump on the bandwagon. We've got to get more people involved. We've got to concentrate on a cure for prostate cancer. That is the key. Most of the new things you hear about and the standard treatments like flutamide and Lupron are not cures. They're all temporary things. We have to keep looking at this thing for a cure."

"To me," said Charlie, "the future of finding a cure for prostate cancer, which I believe is possible, lies in making new discoveries. That depends on having the money to give to the people who make the key finds—and maybe that's the small investigator, not the big organizations. Oftentimes, it's the little guy who gets a grant to follow a line of research that leads to something."

---

*Wall Street Journal*, August 25, 1997.

"I'm sold on what technology can do for us," John added. "I've been in the field of technology almost 50 years, and I know that the potential for a cure is there—the potential is there! Right now our job is to make sure the money is behind us to get that technology moving. An example is the work being done with tumor vaccines by Dr. John Petros at Emory University. We need innovative approaches like this; otherwise every experiment is going to stop dead. We've got to get more people involved. The brainpower is here now! We've got to get these people funded!"

And for John and Charlie, time is of the essence. Both are Stage D2 and running out of options. And sometimes, they say, it's hard not to get discouraged. "We are so far behind," said Charlie, "sometimes I feel as if I'm wasting my time and energy. I'm a management consultant, and if I look at the prostate cancer movement I'd give it a Z in terms of effectiveness. Sometimes it seems very unfocused, scattered, and disconnected."

"It seems like we're basically still back in the '30s," said Paul. "We're really not very far advanced."

It was back in 1930 that researchers from the University of Chicago discovered that removing the testes from animals shut down the production of testosterone. At the same time, researchers also discovered that surgical castration (orchiectomy) could also shrink prostate cancer.*

Then scientists discovered they could do the same thing chemically with female hormones called estrogens. Today, hormonal therapy is successfully helping thousands of men with advanced prostate cancer. But better and more effective treatments are needed—treatments that will impact systemic and metastasized cancer—and that means research must progress. Without awareness, advocacy, and more money, that won't happen.

"As far as advocacy goes," said Peter, "I think one of the directions we need to go is to try and ensure the continued growth of Us Too, Man to Man, PAACT, and all the other support groups."

"Growth and *focus*," added Charlie.

US TOO, Man to Man, and PAACT are the three major support organizations in the United States, and all have chapters scattered

---

*P. C. Walsh, J. F. Worthington, *The Prostate* (Baltimore, MD: Johns Hopkins University Press, 1995).

across the country and internationally. All have undergone growing pains and funding problems. PAACT was started by the late Lloyd Ney and stands independently. US TOO was originally funded by the American Foundation for Urologic Disease (AFUD) but broke away from this organization due to funding and political problems.

"We didn't want to be dominated by a group of doctors who said, 'Our way is the only way,'" commented Rosalie.

Man to Man was founded in 1989 through the committed efforts of a small group of men led by the late Jim Mullen. During the first few years, Man to Man was successful, but the organization was limited on how much it could expand. It was, in fact, looking for a place to call home, and in 1996, Man to Man became a division of the American Cancer Society.

"We had no funds, no staff," recalled Peter, who is president of Man to Man, Inc. in Sarasota, Florida, and a long-time member. "We had maybe 50 chapters, and we said, 'What can we do?' We looked at the ACS. They had 3,400 offices, and they were looking for a prostate cancer arm to go along with their breast cancer program. There were some bumpy places along the way, but it was a logical fit. Otherwise, we could have disappeared or at least stopped growing."

All three organizations currently operate independently from each other, and all wish to continue their autonomy. Although there are operating differences among them and at times political rivalry, there's really not a whole lot that separates them philosophically.

"What we need, too," said John, "is some type of agreement between us. We need to open up the lines of communication between the three organizations." (John is one of the directors of US TOO.) "We are in the business of helping people and we need to work together. We don't want to and we don't need to get involved in the politics of the different organizations, where somebody is going to dictate to us, and I don't think you want anybody dictating to your organizations. I am well aware of the fact that we've done an extremely poor job as far as raising money. We've gotten some grants of $50,000 and $60,000 and we've gotten some for over $100,000, but that's nickels and dimes. At the US TOO offices in Hinsdale, Illinois, our monthly bill runs into the thousands of dollars because we've got an 800 number. We feel it's well worth spending that money because our job is to help people like ourselves, and that's exactly what we're doing—helping people. PAACT has this in mind, and Peter (Man to Man) has this is mind. This is why we must come to a meeting of the minds. We're all in this together, and if we're going to raise money—and raise big money—we cannot compete with ourselves."

Charlie is PAACT's liaison to US TOO International and is working to bring PAACT and US TOO closer together. "If we could just get together, what could we do?" he asked. "US TOO has approximately 100,000 members. PAACT has 33,000 members. The funding gap between breast cancer and prostate cancer in federal grants is about $420 million a year. Could we form an organization that would bridge the gap of $420 million a year, and how long would it take? Can we do a better job of communicating to cancer patients and patients-to-be? The job is enormous. If we are going to do something really significant with prostate cancer, we are going to have to mount an offensive of unselfishness, size, and commitment that transcends what we have ever done before. 'United we stand. Divided we fall.'"

"Our support group in Portland is independent from all of you," said Paul. "If you want to be US TOO or whatever, come on in. We don't have any problem with that, and as far as I know we don't follow any particular agenda. If there's going to be a coalition, these independent support groups should also be tied together to develop a political action committee that could have some thrust."

"Our support group in Albuquerque," said Derek, "is also independent. We organize free prostate cancer screenings every year with the cooperation of the hospitals and are going straight to the state and federal governments for assistance in funding. Like Rosalie, we feel that we didn't want to be controlled by doctors. We greatly appreciate those who assist us but find many of them pretty narrow-minded in their treatment options and advice to patients."

"I've talked with doctors who have said that all the support groups could and should be doing much more than we are," added Peter. "If we can get to a congressperson or senator, and if he or she gets eight letters on an issue, that sparks their attention. That's the break point, the magic number. And it isn't the Senator Dole-type person who's too big and has too many issues. We need to find a person who doesn't have a cause yet. And you can't argue with a cause of federal funding for prostate cancer. It's a great cause, so if you can find someone who hasn't got a bandwagon

Virgil's prostate website:
http://www.prostate-online.com
The Prostate Net
P.O. Box 2192
Secaucus, NJ 07096
1–888–4-PROSNET
vhsimons@pipeline.com

yet, or several people, and get them to submit the bills, maybe that's the way to go."

Whether it's eight-plus letters to your representative or a march on Washington, there is, undeniably, strength and power en masse. However, individual efforts in prostate cancer advocacy (and there are thousands of men and women across the country volunteering their time) are creating and perpetuating their own strong ripple effects. Virgil is mounting his own tsunami wave.

"I feel I have to do something," he told us. "I can't sit around and just talk about it, and I've committed myself to the fight in doing what I can. We are going after the state-elected officials of New York, specifically Governor Pataki, to have him sponsor a bill in the New York state assembly that will mandate reimbursement of prostate cancer screening. There had been an effort this past session, but it died. What I did was go on the Internet and post to all the major news groups and forums the e-mail addresses of key legislators, the governor, and other key federal people. Unfortunately, the timing was such that they just couldn't get the bill passed this session. But the response was so incredible. People sat up and took notice, to the point I'm presenting a plan to a major pharmaceutical company to get them to develop a whole Internet lobbying arm. That way we can use the Internet to get behind lobbying, state by state, national or whatever.

"I've also set up an alliance with part of the Hispanic community in and around the New York area. I'm working on prostate cancer segments for various TV shows, and I'm going after *Ebony* magazine, *Black Enterprise,* and *Essence* to start doing articles on prostate cancer as it relates to the black community. Concurrently, I'm going after every one of the computer magazines to present the issue of health care maintenance and controlling your own health via the Internet—and suggesting that they tie in the prostate cancer imperative. I've also got proposals into the local network affiliates to talk about using the Internet as a way of dealing with prostate cancer, and I'm using myself as an example. I've got a website going and I've written a brochure and the *On-line Guide to Fighting Prostate Cancer,* which you can use in conjunction with your health care provider. Both are designed to help you take an active role in your health care.

"I think one of the most worthwhile things I've done is produce a consultation form that patients can take with them when they go to the doctor. It has a whole range of topics to discuss and what it does is force the individual to think about what he's got, to understand it, and make informed decisions. It helps patients talk with their doctor and it helps the doctor talk with the patient.

"I've also put together a magazine insert planned for *Forbes* which will give a major editorial focus to prostate cancer. The reason I'm going with *Forbes* is that I want to reach the CEOs of major corporations and get them plugged into the movement. If you get the 'money' out there saying, 'Hey, we're doing something in September about prostate cancer. Can I count on your company to be a part of it?' it opens the door for other things. I can't be involved in egos. We've got to save lives! If we can do it together, great, but I'm not going to stand by and wait for all the support groups to get their act together."

"I've listened to Virgil, and I'm very excited about what he's doing," answered Charlie. "I think that's great. But instead of doing what you're doing as individual Virgils, why not do it as part of PAACT plus US TOO? With all that energy and those great ideas, you would automatically have 130,000 people behind you."

"Let's just see if there's a way we can work together," challenged John. "There are areas where Man to Man is ahead of US TOO, where PAACT is ahead of US TOO. If we can concentrate on our individual specialties and work together, that would be the beginning. There are a lot of misconceptions and rumors going on because of past histories and I say, 'Let's clean off the table.' I'll put you on our mailing list [US TOO's]; you fellas get information that we don't get. I'm sure we're getting information that you don't get. I don't care. I get up at meetings and tell them this information came from PAACT or Man to Man. It doesn't matter to me.

"If we don't communicate," John concluded, "we're not reaching the thousands of people out there that know nothing about support groups."

We have a long way to go. Perhaps even a longer journey in reaching the traditionally medically underserved populations. There is a disproportionate incidence of cancer mortality among minorities and persons of lower socioeconomic status for many reasons including lack of awareness, diet, religious or cultural beliefs, no insurance, and transportation problems. For unknown reasons, African Americans suffer the highest incidence of prostate cancer in the world and also have the highest rate of death.

"You look at the black and Hispanic communities," began Virgil, "and to an extent, macho is very important. You're not going to be able to say to a guy, 'Hey, maybe there's something wrong with your Johnson.' He's not going to deal with it—he just won't even brook the potential of it. Those kind of filters, artificial or whatever, inhibit people from even recognizing a potential problem, much less dealing with a problem when they get it.

"For example, I've tried to talk an Hispanic couple into coming to support groups. They won't come. The guy says, 'Virg, I can't stand up there and let people know about my problem!' I said, 'But your problem is not going to go away.'"

"We have problems reaching people, too," said John. "We've been trying to get African Americans to be part of our US TOO group. We've gone to churches where the minister has made special arrangements for us to go in. But you only get from two to five people show up. You go into other places, and we've gone to some of the biggest churches in Chicago—black churches—and you just don't get a turnout. One of our support group members is black, and he's gone to these places, and he's been trying to teach us what to do and what to say, and we've tried. We've gone into the neighborhoods, their storefront churches, and we just don't know what to do anymore."

"That doesn't just apply to black people," observed Paul. "It applies to our whole civilization. I don't think anybody is really interested until they get the problem."

"I know people who have Ph.D.'s," said Bob, "and they refuse to read anything about prostate cancer. After a diagnosis, they will not go back to their doctors. They just ignore the problem. You talk about watchful waiting!"

"A lot of people, too," said Paul, "are just not skilled in reading or exchanging information or playing on computers, and I think we should try and reach these people and tell them, 'Hey, you don't have to read anything, all you have to do is come to a support group and we'll tell you if you can't read.' Unfortunately, we don't get to those people."

"That's why we need to get to the doctors," Derek emphasized. "The doctors need to immediately refer their patients to support groups. They need to say, 'You've got prostate cancer. Now go to a support group; take your time to learn about all your choices.' Support groups need the doctors' cooperation to get these newly diagnosed men early. The doctors need our cooperation to get patients—and they'll have better, informed patients."

"You also have people whose family doctor is the emergency room of a hospital," added Virgil. "You've got people who do not as a regular course get regular checkups. You've got people who are systemically fearful of doctors. You have people for a variety of reasons who don't perform the basics of minimal health maintenance. So how do you reach those people who either for lack of interest, lack of education, or lack of motivation don't have the potential to absorb the message?"

It's a tough question. Do we keep trying to reach everybody, or should we just stop trying at some point? Most of us said *No!* and refused to accept the fact that some people can't be helped or won't get the message.

"If we're going to play triage," said Virgil, "then we're saying that certain segments of the population are valuable and others are expendable. We've got to keep trying and we've got to follow through with approaches that work. Sometimes the best intentions are DOA without some careful planning and follow-through and a little common sense thrown in. For example, take free screening. Free screening is wonderful if you know that it's happening. I was talking to a guy in my support group who says, 'It's being advertised on the radio station.' Well, if you don't listen to that radio station, you aren't going to know that the screening is taking place. Making it available is one thing, but you've got to be able to get the message out in a broad enough way, in the various media that people can really access and understand."

"But what is that medium?" asked Bob.

"If nothing else," said Virgil, "I believe you ought to get companies like Budweiser on board. On every six-pack, you start promoting the idea of prostate cancer awareness. Hey, why not? You've got couch potatoes out there. If the guy's only involvement is the TV and the six-pack, then put the message on the goddamn six-pack!"

"Which is exactly what the women's groups have done with breast cancer," said Bob. "You look at the numbers of people who are aware of that now. You see breast cancer awareness messages everywhere."

"One of the best examples for breast cancer awareness is four of the major manufacturers of brassieres got together to promote Breast Cancer Awareness Month," added Virgil. "In every package of brassieres, they were putting a little message about breast cancer awareness, self-testing, and all of that. That's the kind of thing we should be doing."

"It's the same with heart attacks and heart disease," said Manuel. "It seemed like we once had an epidemic of heart attacks. Now they seem to be decreasing with more awareness about the importance of diet and recognizing the warning signs."

Or, as Bud put it, "Maybe you have to use the ole farm boy's approach. Remember the saying 'You can lead a horse to water but you can't make him drink'? A lot of people didn't realize you could put salt in his oats, and that's what I'm saying we've got to do. You've got to give them something to go to, to want to receive it."

"Just remember, said Charlie, "that the money gap is $420 million a year as we speak in federal grants for research. That is so important, and it's why I come back to it over and over again."

## The National Prostate Cancer Coalition

When all of us met at this retreat in summer 1996, the National Prostate Cancer Coalition (NPCC) was in its embryonic phase. Growing pains were evident as the coalition devised its organizational structure and determined its focus and course of action.

Despite political differences, this effort brought together the first broad-based coalition to address prostate cancer issues with survivors, families, advocates, researchers, physicians, and manufacturers and created a simple but powerful mission: the elimination of prostate cancer as a disease of serious concern for men and their families.

> With millions of federal research dollars at stake, the National Prostate Cancer Coalition is calling on the American people to insist on appropriate funding for prostate cancer. You can get involved in advocacy work by
>
> - calling or writing your representatives and senators,
> - calling the NPCC,
> - contacting your local support group or the national offices of Man to Man, PAACT, and US TOO, International. (See Chapter 2 for more information on support groups.)
>
> The National Prostate Cancer Coalition
> 1156 15th NW, Suite 905
> Washington, D.C. 20005
> 202–463–9455
> http://rattler.cameron.edu/npcc

The coalition has developed an agenda that includes mobilizing human and fiscal resources to increase prostate cancer research, advocating for legislative and regulatory changes that will benefit patients and families, and focusing public awareness on the key issues regarding prevention, diagnosis, and treatment of prostate cancer.

It launched this outreach effort with a massive petition drive to collect 1 million signatures in support of additional funding for prostate cancer. Those signatures will be delivered to Capitol Hill to capture the attention of Washington and those individuals who control key budget decisions.

Before we move on, there are some vitally important topics that need revisiting: awareness, prevention, and early detection. Some of us at this retreat, including Derek, Manuel, Virgil, and Bob, were extremely fortunate because our cancer was diagnosed early, when it was still confined to the capsule. With urgent prompting by some of the wives, as you'll remember, we took the initiative and underwent the digital rectal exam and the PSA test.

The point is, they took some preventative action. And that is what we want all men to do. Beginning at age 40, or earlier if you have a family history of prostate cancer or breast cancer (men in families with breast cancer are at an increased risk for developing prostate cancer), ask your doctor to perform a DRE. Remember, you may

---

## Research Update

According to the American Cancer Society, many critical research questions remain to be addressed, including the following:

- How known prostate cancer risk factors influence the age at which screening should be started.
- The influence of patient characteristics, risk factors, and previous test outcomes on PSA screening intervals.
- The psychosocial impact of screening.
- Cost-effectiveness and different strategies for the efficient delivery of screening to yield the most cost-effective medical care.
- Enhancements of PSA testing including density, velocity, doubling time, form, and age-specific and race-specific PSA.
- New tests that may complement or serve as alternatives to PSA, and tests that may predict the aggressiveness of disease; among these new tests are prostate-specific membrane antigen and prostate markers in other body fluids (such as seminal fluid, urine, saliva).
- New imaging and biopsy techniques.

Source: A. von Eschenbach, R. Ho, G. P. Murphy, M. Cunningham, N. Lins. American Cancer Society guideline for the early detection of prostate cancer: Update 1997. *CA: A Cancer Journal for Clinicians* 47 (1997):261–264.

---

need to be proactive and ask for it if your doctor doesn't suggest it. Ask your doctor about the PSA test. If you want the test, have it performed. Inform yourself about prostate cancer *before* you need the information. That way, if you are diagnosed, you'll already have some basic knowledge. It probably won't lessen the shock of a diagnosis; nothing can prepare you for that. But at least you'll be armed with some information that may help lessen the initial fear of this disease. And then, as all of us would recommend, head for the nearest support group—online, in-person, or both.

## Lifelines: Resources and the Internet

"Computers are great," said Charlie, "and I love what I can do with mine. But a support group is a bunch of human beings, and a support group is never the same as the *Encyclopedia Brittanica*. The In-

# Research Update

The rapid rise in the incidence of prostate cancer between the years 1988 and 1992 has been attributed to prostate-specific antigen (PSA) screening.

A recent study analyzed prostate cancer screening in the United States using 208,234 prostate cancer cases diagnosed between 1973 and 1993 in population-based Surveillance, Epidemiology, and End Results (SEER) registries. The study says that the dramatic spike in incidence of prostate cancer is greater than has ever been recorded for any cancer.

The study went on to say that two conditions must be met to have a successful screening program. First, there must be a test or procedure that can detect cancers earlier. Second, earlier treatment must result in a better outcome. The screening tests must also be able to create lead time, that is, to detect malignancies in asymptomatic individuals.

In prostate cancer, screening tests are primarily composed of a PSA test in combination with a digital rectal exam (DRE). The results of the study showed that after the PSA test was introduced in the late 1980s a rapid increase in incidence of the disease occurred between 1988 and 1993, reaching a zenith in 1992 and then declining. This pattern fits a screening phenomenon. The major increase in incidence was observed in patients with early-stage disease that would have otherwise been diagnosed at a later time. There was a decrease in the rate and number of patients detected with advanced disease, as expected.

A decrease in deaths from prostate cancer is the ultimate goal of screening. In November 1996, a preliminary report from the National Center for Health Statistics noted a 11.2 percent decrease in the U.S. mortality rate for prostate cancer between 1991 and 1995.

The SEER data from 1973–1993 demonstrated all the criteria of a successful screening program. Data suggest that screening reduces the incidence of advanced disease, which influences the mortality rate. Based on these data, the study concluded that there should be no change in the present guidelines recommending an annual PSA blood test and a DRE for all men 50 years and over with a life expectancy of greater than ten years.

Source: C. R. Smart. The results of prostate carcinoma screening in the U.S. as reflected in the surveillance, epidemiology, and end results program. *Cancer* 80 (1997):1835–1844.

ternet is a different animal. It is so huge. The amount of information is mind-boggling. But a human being can respond to you more directly, instantaneously, and in many ways more compassionately and more effectively than a computer. So I would never say that a support group in any way would be replaced by a computer."

"And I agree with that," said Virgil. "I attend three support groups. I'm not just one of those people who just sit at a computer. But you have to keep in mind that most support groups only meet once a month. If you can't get to a support group, where do you go for help?"

"I think that the computer and support groups go hand in hand," said Paul. "They complement each other. But I do think that when you make eye contact with somebody, that's very special."

"No question," answered Virgil, "but I disagree that the Internet lacks a face-to-face content. You find that in the course of a dialogue, through either the bulletin boards or the forums, you really get a chance to express what you feel, get to the heart of the issue, and it's not colored by artificial things. You're able to really talk about your feelings and have them come through."

"The Internet is good for those comfortable with it," countered Charlie, "but a lot of people just feel better communicating in person at a support group or hearing someone's voice over the phone. It's what works best for you."

If you have the option, take advantage of every kind of support you can find, because emotional bonds and friendships can be forged in any setting. In fact, Virgil and Manuel met on the Internet in 1994. They maintained a frequent dialogue of their daily battles and victories with this disease and became an incredible source of support for each other. They met in person for the first time at this retreat. Hugging each other when they arrived, they looked like old friends reuniting. And in fact, they were.

If you haven't already guessed, Virgil was our resident Internet guru, and he was more than happy to share his expertise. During one of our sessions, we were treated to an online seminar with Virgil at his laptop. We watched and listened as he guided us through the ins and outs of going online.

"It's funny," said Virgil. "When we were younger we would talk about how big our tools were, and then how big our cars were and how fast they were. Now, as we've gotten older, we talk about who's got the biggest hard drive. The toys have just changed.

"One of the wonderful things is e-mail, or the ability to transmit your messages electronically. This is probably one of the most important things because the world is opened up to you. Right now I'm looking at messages from people from the West Coast to the East Coast and from Australia to Austria. You're able to communicate literally with the whole world for a very small cost—basically a local phone call. It's an extended support network. I have people log onto my website, leave messages that say, 'I need help. I need somebody to talk to.' These are often guys who don't have support groups near them or don't really know how to go about getting support. It's a way of extending the range of our involvement to help others."

"The Internet is going to play a big part in our health care," said John, "simply because information is on the machine much sooner than it can be by word of mouth or by mail. And the people I've talked to on the Internet are more than pleased. We've gotten stacks of literature and information at US TOO from people who've gotten it off the computer. But you have to realize that there are many people in the older age group that do not have a computer, and they're not channeling their thinking towards that. It's tunnel vision, and there's a little tunnel vision among all of us."

"Some people just aren't interested in computers," offered Charlie. "For some people it becomes a hobby, just like a hobby of piano playing or growing flowers. If you don't care about getting information and using a computer, you're not going to be interested in the Internet. The Internet is incredibly valuable to me, and I've gotten tremendous information off of it. But I'm very computer literate, and I'm totally involved with it in my business as well. And I agree with John. The Internet is the wave of the future."

"I am one of those computer illiterates," admitted Bob. "After I left the police department, I swore I'd never use a computer for anything. Well, I recently bought one, and a desk to put it in, and it should be installed in about a week or two. Then I have to get an e-mail address. So I guess the message is, never say never."

Virgil continued with his online seminar. "Besides e-mail there's another wonderful thing you can get called a newsgroup. A newsgroup is a forum where people come together around a specific topic, in this case it's prostate cancer, but it could be gardening or sailing or legal issues. There are thousands of topics out there. People from around the world will post to this newsgroup and help each other out in any way they can. For example, there's a doctor

who talks about lessons learned from breast cancer and about sharing them with the group. Men talk about any and all elements of
prostate cancer, be it sexual problems, diagnosis and treatments,
and where to find information on the topic. People post a message,
everybody will read it, and anybody can respond to it and give their
input. So it's not unlike the give-and-take we have here physically at
this retreat, only it takes place over the Net. You lack a little of the
immediacy, but the thread of the messages are held together. Anything you want to know, anything you feel comfortable talking
about, you can talk about it here and the world can respond. I've
had people give me input from as far away as Beijing, China.
There's a doctor of philosophy there who has prostate cancer. He
said, 'I saw your web page, let's talk about this,' and we exchanged
information on herbal therapies. It's this kind of universal experience that we need to plug in to."

"And there's another advantage to being online," said Manuel.
"You can be anonymous or as open as you want. At first, Virgil and
I didn't know anything about each other except each other's names.
Then, after a while we started feeling more comfortable, and we ex-
changed telephone numbers."

If you're interested in venturing online, here are some basics.
First, you have to have what's called "online services." Those are
companies like America Online, Compuserve, Microsoft Network,
and Prodigy, and their intent is to provide a self-contained universe
of information. As a component, they have access to the Internet,
but they primarily want you to stay within the confines of that online service. You pay a monthly fee for the right to be a member of
the service. If you go into the premium forums, like the cancer forums, you'll pay an additional hourly charge.

"The other vehicle of access is what's called an Internet service
provider," said Virgil. "This could be a national or local company
that gives you direct access to the Internet. It's the doorway you
walk through. Usually, you'll pay a flat fee for unlimited hours per
month. For example, the one I use is $19.95 a month and I can stay
on there as many hours as I want. On some other services it's very
easy to run up bills in excess of $80, $90, $100 a month or more be-
cause of additional charges that can accrue. So to sum this all up,
the information contained in an online service is only what it physically has within its network, whereas if you access the Internet—the
world is yours!"

---

### Search Engines

Search.Com
   http://www.search.com
Yahoo
   http://www.yahoo.com
Alta Vista
   http://www.altavista.digital.com

---

So once you've got access to the Internet, how do you find your way around? As Paul pointed out, "There's such a huge volume of information out there, it's difficult to get a handle on it." It can be a little overwhelming at first, but once you've narrowed down what you want to know, you can use what's called a search engine to help you find specific information from all the available databases on the web.

"I use a search tool called Search.Com—that's http://www.search.com," said Virgil. "It's 300 different search engines all located on one page. If you're interested in the arts, there are search engines that will take you there. If you're into automotive, there are search engines that will take you there. If you want information about prostate cancer, there are any number of ways to get there. In my opinion one of the best is a search engine called Yahoo. It provides one of the strongest databases on health information out there. You can scroll down to health, and under health you'll find a whole range of things. Click on diseases, and it will take you to the next hierarchy of information, which will give you another range of choices. Alta Vista is another excellent search tool that divides the web into broad subject areas including cancer and prostate cancer, specifically."

However you get your information, our message to you is *get it*! And if you are so motivated, and we hope that you are, get involved with your local support group or the NPCC and call and write your elected officials and make your individual voice heard. Without a strong, united, and sustained effort, we will not find better treatments for this disease. We will not find a cure.

As we said at the beginning of this chapter, we are advocates. And we are fighting not only for our own lives and the lives of all men affected by this disease but for our sons and our grandsons. It was

# Information Services

The National Cancer Institute (NCI) sponsors the Physician Data Query (PDQ), a computerized listing of up-to-date cancer information for health professionals and patients on the latest types of cancer treatments and clinical studies testing new and promising cancer treatments. PDQ is accessible through several NCI-sponsored services, including

- CancerFax—CancerFax is a service that provides cancer information by fax. To use CancerFax, dial 301–402–5874 from the telephone on a fax machine and listen to the recorded instructions to receive a faxed CancerFax contents list.
- CancerNet—CancerNet is a service through which cancer information can be obtained by computer. CancerNet may be accessed using the following methods:
- CancerNet Mail Service (via e-mail)—To obtain the CancerNet contents list, send an e-mail message that says "help" in the body of the message to cancernet@icicc.nci.nih.gov. CancerNet documents can then be ordered through e-mail.
- CancerNet is accessible via the Internet through the World Wide Web (http://cancernet.nci.nih.gov) and Gopher (gopher://gopher.nih.gov) servers.

Other NCI services include

- Cancer Information Service (CIS), a nationwide telephone service providing free information, including referrals to local community cancer resources. Cancer information specialists can answer questions in English or Spanish.
- Numerous publications concerning many aspects of cancer and cancer-related services. Many are available in English or Spanish.

National Cancer Institute
Public Inquiries, Office of Cancer Communication
9000 Rockville Pike
Bethesda, MD 20892
1–800–4-CANCER

For callers with TTY (telecommunications device for deaf persons) equipment: 1–800–332–8615 during our very first dinner together that Bob said, "I came to this retreat to give something back. We're a 'captive' audience here, so by God, let's get together and work to put out an excellent book to help those people who come after us. We are pioneers, and I think we should make a difference."

We hope we have made a difference in your life.

≈≋≈

*"It's late, everyone's tired. Let's call it an evening and reconvene in the morning. Breakfast 7:30–9:00 on the porch . . . thank you all for coming."*

# 1 1

# *Hindsight and Future Visions*
## PHILOSOPHIES REVISITED

*I came to this retreat to learn more about prostate cancer and to give something back. We need to keep learning. We need to keep talking.*
### —Don Zank

*This is like time-lapse photography, like watching the rosebud, and you're going to see a cabbage rose blooming in each of these lives by the time we leave here.*
### —Rosalie Plosnich

## November 1997

All good things must come to an end, or so the saying goes. It's been a little more than a year since we all gathered together at the Graylyn International Conference Center in North Carolina. We came armed with experience and anticipation. We left feeling motivated and excited about this project and with a reinvigorated commitment to helping our fellow human beings. We came with barely a paragraph of information about each other but left with intimate details of each other's lives. We left with friendships just beginning.

Since our time together, we have also lost a friend. John Plosnich died on September 3, 1997. He fought this disease with great vigor, great strength, and style. He was empowered, and, as Charlie observed, "John didn't lose his battle with this disease, because he battled it to the end. It was just his time."

We especially dedicate this book to John, his passion for life, his enthusiasm for this project, and his ever-present hope. "By John

**239**

> From John's Memorial Mass:
>
> ### To Remember Me
>
> *If by chance, you wish to remember me,*
> *do it by giving kindness and compassion*
> *to all you meet.*
> *Show it by the touch of your hand,*
> *by a pat on the back, by a hug, by a kiss.*
> *If you do all I have asked,*
> *I will live forever.*

passing away from the same disease we all are suffering from," said Bob, "it's as if a little of me went with him. I suppose it's from the kinship we shared, even though I only spent five days with him."

And the rest of us? We are all moving forward with our lives.

## Paul Georgeades

My life, it seems, has become an ongoing learning project. Every day there's something new to deal with and new decisions to make.

Fortunately, my PSA remains unmeasurable. For a short amount of time, I switched medications, going from flutamide to bicalutamide, but currently I'm not on any hormonal therapy. However, I'm well aware that there are no guarantees in life and that I can't rely solely on my PSA to predict whether my cancer will return. There are so many other factors involved. But I will continue to have my PSA monitored quarterly and hope that my good fortune sticks around for a while.

The best thing I can do for myself all the way around is to concentrate on good nutrition, sticking to low-fat foods, and try to exercise regularly. Walking is a favorite way to accomplish that, but living out in the rainy Northwest, it's sometimes difficult.

I'm also considering a new therapy that may help restore my sexuality. My doctor has suggested I try a combination of finasteride (Proscar) and DHEA (dehydro-epiandrosterone), which is an adrenal androgen. Interestingly enough, DHEA is currently being sold as an over-the-counter dietary supplement. At one time, you'll remember, I was thinking about taking testosterone shots. Proscar and DHEA may help restore my sexuality without the risks of testosterone. It's worth a try.

If my life has changed in any way, it's that I've become more mellow. Things don't bother me as much as they did even a year ago. Maybe that's because I now have a little better perspective and outlook on life. For example, I'm learning to play the piano. The "old me" would have heaped unreasonable demands on myself. I would have pressured myself to reach a certain goal by a certain date. Today, I just do as much or as little as I want. Life is much more pleasant this way.

If I were to offer a final comment it would be this: It seems to me that most people who are *survivors* and attend support groups are good communicators and leaders. It's up to us as survivors to continue to try to reach out to other men who aren't such good communicators—maybe they can't even read. We need to encourage those men to come to the support groups. If they come, we'll get the information to them.

Finally, as I go through life, I've become more appreciative of things and people who have helped me live through the hard times. I owe a lot to my wife, Phyllis, who dragged me down to the doctor in the first place; to the doctors who treated me and continue to treat me; to the people who make the medicine; and to all the other people behind the scenes. They have all contributed to keeping me alive, and I intend to make the most of it.

## *Aarol (Bud) Irish*

I'm happy to report that my life is normal! I'm off all medications at this point and have a PSA of 1.7, which is a considerable drop since last year. When the book retreat ended in August of 1996, my PSA was 2.6, but it began to rise rapidly. In October it had risen to 5.4, and by November it was 11.275.

In May of 1997 I started on Casodex for approximately 90 days and the trimonthly Lupron shot. Starting Casodex seven days prior to Lupron resulted in fewer hot flashes for me. My latest bone scan in 1997 was negative.

One of the first things I realized at the retreat was that I was not only the oldest but I'd had prostate cancer the longest. Nevertheless, under my treatment regimen of intermittent hormonal therapy, my quality of life has been favorable.

I'm trying to stay healthy by watching what I eat and drink and by staying in shape. I exercise religiously. Every day I lift two five-pound weights 45 times—15 times in three different ways—and try to do 50 "gut busters" a day as well. So far, I've not had any muscle wasting, and I know that my daily exercise has helped prevent that. I still play tennis at least three or four times a week and enjoy golfing, too.

The phones and fax in my home seem to be in constant use and are literally keeping me in touch with hundreds of other prostate cancer survivors. The majority of them report to me how well they're doing with combination hormonal therapy or intermittent therapy, which is great news to me.

I would be remiss not to mention the great relationship as well as friendship, since 1991, with two wonderful people who have been tremendous in providing prostate cancer information—Lloyd Ney, founder of PAACT, and the late Jim Mullen, founder of Man to Man. These two men gave me the greatest support in continuing my treatment. They also kept me traveling across the country from Maine to Alaska, spreading the news about the importance of having annual checkups, especially for early detection, and explaining all of the current treatments. With much humor, in spite of this grim disease, I call them the "captains" and they call me the "messenger."

I used to give several talks a year on prostate cancer around the country, but today, I'm trying to cut back a bit. My advocacy work is extremely important to me, but I also know that I have to have balance in my life. I'm so fortunate that my cancer is in remission and that I can "forget" about having cancer—at least temporarily. In other words, I can walk away from it when I need to and not worry about it in the least. There's so much I enjoy in life, and I enjoy every day to the fullest with my wife, Elaine, and my family.

If I have any words of wisdom I would say to make sure you get a copy of all your tests and keep your records up to date. I could almost write a chapter on errors and changes in tests that I have on record. I would also tell everyone to look in the mirror and say, "I'm going to make it." I believe you become what you think.

I would like to stress that there are good doctors out there with open minds about new treatments and possible cures. Sometimes we come down too hard on the negative side, and we don't see all the good the medical profession has done—and is doing. I hope the information in this book helps both patients and doctors to better understand and accept each other's responses and reactions.

Finally, I would like to thank my doctors in Sarasota, Florida, and their fine staff, who have not only given me a great quality of life without surgery or radiation but have put up with all my requests for copies of my records month by month for the past eight years.

I always say, "I asked God to give me five years." When I left my doctor last, he said to me, "You've made such a crusade of prostate cancer, He will probably give you 20 more." Who knows!

## Charlie Russ

In these last words to you, you'll find me referring to my prostate cancer as Chicago. I've renamed this disease after my hometown and one of the world's greatest cities. Why? Because I once read a book that urged patients to give the disease a friendly, familiar handle so as not to be afraid of it and to deal with it rationally and from an empowered perspective. It sounded like a great idea, and what better name than that of a beautiful, intellectual, and cultural center.

I wish I could tell you that I'm in full remission, but I can't. Unfortunately, Chicago has metastasized to my pelvic bone and has gotten considerably worse since we gathered together last year. My latest bone scan in November 1997 revealed that the cancer is now in my ribs, cervical and thoracic spine, and lungs. My PSA has jumped from 3.2 to 6.2. These latest test results are a shock to me, but I will deal with them. I'm in close contact with my three doctors and nutritionist and am demanding a more aggressive treatment of the metastasis.

But I know this will be difficult. At this stage, I know that medicine can only delay things. After much deliberation, I've decided to try chemotherapy—Novantrone—in hopes of slowing Chicago down. It's a chance I have to take. The irony is, I feel great.

Over the past year, I have changed some of my opinions regarding the medical profession—perhaps softened is a better term. I have come to respect and better appreciate the health care professionals who treat this disease. Without traditional medicine, I would not be alive today.

However, I must emphasize that in talking to large numbers of patients referred to me by PAACT, I've listened to many horror stories about the rush by surgeons to do radical prostatectomies and the failure to explain all treatment options thoroughly. There are, of course, many great doctors who are members of the American Urological Association. Their approach—explaining to their patients what choices are available to them and giving the pluses and minuses of all treatments—should be the benchmark for all physicians.

Unfortunately, there are too many urologists who still have the "hurry up" approach and by habit or design fail to explain in sufficient detail the options that a Chicago patient has and leave the impression that a radical prostatectomy is really the best thing that any patient could select. When you have the knowledge of all treatments available and understand this disease, you are going to be more than a match for the medical professionals, and you'll make the correct decisions about your life. That's the way to maximize your chances of being a true survivor.

To help ensure that you'll be a survivor, I think you also have to have one foot in alternative medicine and one foot in the traditional medical solution. I continue to use alternative treatments. (In fact, at the urging of fellow book contributor Don Zank, I'm now on hydrogen peroxide therapy, too.) They are extremely important to me, but they are adjuncts, complementing my more traditional treatments. The same with nutrition. I became a vegetarian, and that, I believe, has helped keep me alive. Just as important, good nutrition has given me something to focus on and the power and energy to keep going.

I think that we also have to keep in mind that doctors are not trained in complementary or alternative therapies. There are no studies proving or disproving their effectiveness, and there's no consistency with them. Doctors can't prescribe them, and they're not comfortable suggesting them. That is where the empowered patient comes in. He must search out these alternative choices and, if he sees fit, use them (with his doctor's knowledge) in combination with traditional medicine—or alone. That is his choice.

In some ways, all treatments are alternative because there is no cure for this disease. Each man reacts differently. And in fact, it often seems that traditional medicine can be just as anecdotal as alternative medicine. Think of the high failure rate and recurrence statistics with radiation and also with radical prostatectomies. Think of the prescribed drugs that don't work. To sum up, alternative needs conventional medicine and vice versa. It's like love and marriage.

One thing that has remained constant is my passion for knowledge and for keeping pace with the ever-changing information about
this disease. I call the process "forever learning." I have also found
that the real battle of prostate cancer is within myself. During this
past year, I have faced my own mortality and that has been tough—
particularly after fighting this disease so hard for six years. It has
also been scary. I call it "hitting the wall." But, lo and behold, I
bounced off that wall, perhaps a bit bruised and shaken but ready
to carry on—wherever that leads.

I'm still heavily involved with PAACT and LAC-PAACT, which
has given me a unique experience, to say the least. We're still at war
with Medicare and the Health Care Financing Administration
(HCFA) and encouraging litigation when health care claims are denied. However, I'm making a major effort to let go of a lot of things
and disengage myself from many of the organizations of which I
love to be a part. I feel that it was a healthy thing for me to do. I'm
much more mellow, if you can believe that (believe it), and happier.

One of the things I will treasure most from our gathering is that I
met some really great people with whom I shared a lot and learned a
lot. They have become important members of my support team. It
took a long time for me to appreciate the incredible value of having
a really excellent support group team, and it doesn't have to be
large. A small handful of people of quality are worth ten times more
than an army of those who don't know up from down or don't care
about you. Likewise, there are family members who can be support
people and family members who love you but don't have the knowledge to help you or have trouble communicating with you because
they don't know what to do.

Your support people don't necessarily have to live in your city to
be effective either. My number one support person is Don Zank. He
lives hundreds of miles from Kansas City, but I talk to him virtually
every week—and his wife, Lynne, too.

So despite the trauma associated with Chicago, it's an ill wind
that's blown a lot of good. I'm ready to face whatever happens.
Prayer and a reinforced and more focused understanding of life
have caused me to see that no matter what happens, there is no de-
feat, only victory.

Finally, the search and the energy it takes to maintain my empowerment has kept my notorious enthusiasm at its interstellar level and
helped me survive with a chance for remission way past what my

doctors have predicted. In short, I'm not healthy, but I'm not sick either. Maintaining that level is what it's all about, and if you do, you'll have a much better chance of reaching the ultimate goal of remission regardless of what stage disease you have. That's real health and the key to success and survivorship.

So good hunting to you all. If you keep your head screwed on straight, you can face anything. Even if you had an Olympic body but lost your mental health, you would be totally lost. So keep your mind on the ball, and you'll take care of your body.

## Virgil Simons

I am happy to say that my health remains excellent. My PSA is still less than 0.01. I feel that my battle against prostate cancer has been fought to a draw and that I'll have won only if I die of something else. Having said that, I no longer think about dying. I really focus on the moment. In fact, I've stopped wearing a watch because time in the future has no meaning. Only what I'm doing with the time I'm experiencing now matters.

I still use a lot of herbal and natural therapies and am focusing more on plain, healthy living, although I'm not getting as much rest or exercise as I should because I'm involved in so many projects. But I feel energized by it all!!

I'm in the process of launching a nonprofit organization and getting all the funding in place for that. It also looks as if we're pretty well locked for a prostate cancer article in *Forbes* magazine for September 1999, plus a joint consumer retail program. I've been working on some local and national television programs, and I'm also involved with some of the federal agencies on newly established committees. I'm very excited to report that I've been selected to sit on the Department of Defense's Peer Review Research Panel.

What last advice would I give? Know that doctors can be good or bad and you can no longer make assumptions as to their competence or capability. I've learned to question every one of them regardless of whether the question has to do with prostate cancer or a muscle strain. I've just become a lot more educated about my health and treatments all the way around.

And as much as we stress awareness and early detection and regular screening, a far more important issue is "compliance"—what do you do with the knowledge gained? Too many men are still engaged in the denial of death and either don't want to get tested because of what may be found or, if they do get tested, don't want to deal with the results and necessary follow-up. This is where we must involve family, friends, community, and corporations to encourage that compliance in any way we can.

My work has just begun.

## Peter Stults

Generally speaking, I'm very healthy, which is probably the best news I can give you. Since the retreat, and after 53 months on combination hormonal therapy, I made the decision to try intermittent hormonal therapy. I began IHT in October of 1997, and so far my monthly PSAs have remained unmeasurable. As we all know, however, that could change. My next few tests will be crucial, and my doctor and I will be watching them very carefully.

I've also added selenium to my treatment regimen—250mg a day—but that's about it for changes in treatment. I am trying to exercise more and eat better, which is always a struggle, but I've lost ten pounds since the retreat, and I'm feeling good.

Prostate cancer is a part of my life, and living with it over the years has affected me and my family in many different ways. That's just the way it is. The fact that I have this disease can't be changed, and you learn to deal with the surprising twists and turns that this disease throws out and sometimes precipitates. You learn to deal with them or you don't survive.

Fortunately, I'm feeling at least as comfortable with my disease as I did at the retreat. I'm still president of Man to Man Inc. in Sarasota, and I've been talking a lot more with newly diagnosed patients who call for advice. They're hungry for information, and because their doctors usually want to move quickly, they say it's nice to have someone with whom they can discuss options. Clearly, I feel I'm helping these men deal with their diagnosis and put it into some perspective. Talking to them also continues to help me deal with my own disease.

The advice I give them is what all of us emphasized at the retreat. You must learn as much as you can about this disease. Take charge of your own health. Your doctor is your consultant, but you make the final decisions. Keeping a positive attitude is at least as important. I can't stress that enough.

What's in my future? I'm obviously hoping IHT works for me. The chemicals are slowly working their way out of my body. So we'll see what happens. Change is inevitable, and I will be ready for anything that comes my way.

## Manuel Vazquez

First of all, I'm very fortunate to tell you that there have been no changes in my health since the retreat. My PSA has remained unde-tectable for more than three years now, and for that I am grateful.

Some of my thoughts about life, however, have changed and I'd like to share these with you. After much soul-searching, I have discarded many naive thought patterns in order to come to this conclusion: Evil comes in two flavors. One is the evil you bring upon your-self through self-destructive behaviors; these behaviors have consequences that are easy to foresee. There is also random evil, such as inherited genetic traits or being in the wrong place at the wrong time. This expression of evil is the most difficult to deal with.

Many of us have been conditioned through our moral upbringing to think about bad things as "justified punishment" for our own de-liberate actions. It would have been a lot easier for me to accept my sexual impotency had I done something to bring it about.

I have just let all my anger hang out. Anger is a very valid human feeling, and I am not ashamed to make it known exactly how I feel. However, I have learned to channel the negative energy associated with uncontrollable anger into being a positive force in advocacy and into counseling my fellow prostate cancer patients. I'm also excited to report that I've been selected to be an advocate reviewer for the Prostate Cancer Research Program of the Department of Defense.

Throughout it all I have survived, and I have learned how to live with prostate cancer. I can now use my experiences to guide a newly diagnosed patient in truth and sincerity, and with empathy, through what will probably be the most difficult time in his life. However, I would like to emphasize that there are as many coping mechanisms as there are patients. At one time, I was so enraged that I thought I was losing my mind. With time and with my wonderful, understanding wife, Mary, psychological healing is most definitely taking place.

I am continuing to try anything and everything to restore my sex-uality, but everything has thus far failed. Presently, I am waiting for

FDA approval of sildenafil (Viagra), a new oral medication. The last resort is an implant, but since this would forever alter my anatomy, I would not make that final decision lightly.

I continue to take antioxidants regularly; stay away from fats, primarily animal fats; and consume high quantities of fruits, vegetables, and whole-grain cereals.

We talked a lot about doctors at the retreat and the medical profession in general. Since the retreat, my basic philosophy regarding doctors has not changed much. I believe that overall, doctors are sincere "professionals" who believe wholeheartedly in the training and disciplines passed on to them. However, I put quotation marks around the word professional to indicate a basic flaw in Western medicine. A "professional" is often cold, detached, aloof, and treats people as if they were in vitro specimens. If these "professionals" could only get a temporary case of the disease they treat, their behavior would be radically different. I am not a tumor. I am a person.

I would love for all of the professionals to see the movie *The Doctor*. There are some fellow survivors in my support group who happen to be doctors and specialists in their fields, and their behavior now is probably totally different than it was when they were just "specialists." This is likely one of the reasons patients are flocking to alternative therapies—to fill the void in their treatment.

Finally, I wish to say that I got a lot of satisfaction participating in the retreat. I learned to love all those nine guys and their wives. If I help just one reader of this book, the entire project will have been worthwhile.

Life goes on, and it is worth living even if there is a price to pay to stay alive. My best advice to all is to share your feelings. Don't clam up. If you do, you will pay dearly for it.

## Bob White

The five days spent at the book retreat in North Carolina was an experience that I will treasure the rest of my life. The camaraderie, the sharing of information, and the fact that we were bound by a common bond even though we were from different walks of life, different ethnicities, and different religious beliefs caused me to realize how much alike we all were.

Often I think of those of us whose religious beliefs were shaken and those who felt as though God had played a cruel joke on them and discarded all religious ties. My religious beliefs remain intact, although I can now understand how one could possibly adopt another viewpoint.

At this time, I believe I was fortunate in my choice of treatment. According to Lewis and Berger's book entitled *New Guidelines for Surviving Prostate Cancer*, seed implants will become the "gold standard" in treatment by the year 2000. I suggest every prostate cancer patient read this book. As of this writing, I am entering my fifth year since diagnosis and my third year since having seeds implanted. Bill Dehn, one of the founders of my prostate cancer support group in Fullerton, California (the Prostate Forum), is a 12-year survivor, a fact that heavily influenced my choice of treatment. Before treatment, my PSA was 8.5. Now it hovers in the vicinity of 0.38 with no side effects as a result of the implants.

My outlook for the future as far as prostate cancer is concerned is bright; however, my concern is now focused on a new problem that has arisen. In August of 1996, right after the book retreat, I was diagnosed with non-Hodgkin's lymphoma. In September of the same year, a malignant tumor was removed from the left side of my neck. Since then, I have had bone scans, CAT scans, and bloodwork at four-month intervals. So far, all are negative (thank God!). My doctor told me the same thing my urologist told me about prostate cancer. "Whatever is going to take you away from here, it's not going to be this!" Needless to say, I am not just lucky. I am very blessed!

I now belong to two support groups, learning all I can about these diseases, helping others, and maintaining a very positive outlook on life. I recommend reading, laughing, loving, music, art, smelling the flowers, praying and giving thanks for those whom you love and who love you. Tomorrow is not promised, but you can certainly enjoy today.

God bless.

### *Derek Workman*

In the year that's passed since the gathering of "the Gang at Graylyn" a few things have happened that I'd like to share.

With regard to my health, my PSA has continued to rise slowly and steadily and that has really worn on my mind. You don't forget about this thing—EVER! At least I don't.

Finally, in August of 1997, I contacted the Education Center for Prostate Cancer Patients founded by Dr. James Lewis and Dr. E.

Roy Berger, and they told me about testing being done at the University of California at San Francisco with spectroscopic MRI.

After I had this test, the doctors thought I had a recurrence in the prostate but saw nothing in the surrounding bone area or lymph system. I immediately followed that news with a trip to see Dr. Fred Lee at Crittenton Hospital in Rochester, Michigan, for an ultrasound and eight biopsies.

I got the results the following day. Dr. Lee told me that there was NO CANCER and "certainly no cancer in your prostate." Finally, some good news! Ramona, my significant other, and I celebrated. Dr. Lee said that the probable explanation of my rising PSA is possible regrowth of healthy prostate cells and that my PSA should stabilize soon. We'll be watching it and hoping that it stops its damned climb in the coming year. I plan to stay "off" all therapies unless my PSA goes above 2.0. If that happens, we'll take a look at additional therapies.

At this point, I'm moving toward an even stronger positive position on hormonal therapy. Intermittent hormonal therapy and triple hormone blockade tests are showing some wonderful results, including an improved quality of life. Some men I know have been on a particular combined hormonal therapy for one year and have been "off" for up to four years and are still counting. So, for these men at least, it seems to be very effective, and I'm very interested in it if I should at some point need additional therapy.

We're trying to continue to contact more guys in the area to let them know about our support group. But we've got to do more, by whatever means, to get the newly diagnosed patients to the support groups before they get talked into something that they may not want or need. I feel that the amount of damage still being done is completely unacceptable. Fortunately, I think we are slowly winning over doctors to the idea that newly diagnosed patients should contact a support group as soon as possible.

The march goes on to help as many as we can.

### Don Zank

First and foremost I'd like to thank my wife, Lynne, for her unconditional support. I know I could never have started and maintained my program of alternative therapies without her.

Second, I'd like to emphasize that because of my therapy choices, I still have all my body parts, and they still function. I'm also glad to report that my health status is the same, which is excellent! I'm still on the same alternative program as before, and I haven't started any new therapies.

To be honest, I'm probably more antidoctor and traditional medicine than I was at the retreat. I believe that greed is running the medical profession. It seems that no one wants to seriously look at alternative therapies, which have afforded me a decent life without the side effects. They're simply being dismissed, and that's too bad.

That's why *you must do your homework before you choose your treatment!* I feel that I made the right choice for Don Zank, and I will live and die with my choice.

I believe that anyone diagnosed with prostate cancer should not make a snap decision. It probably took several years for the cancer to develop. In most cases, you can take some time to research both the disease and the many treatments available.

If you're interested in alternative therapies, there *is* information out there. You'll find a lot on the Internet. You'll also want to join PAACT and get its newsletter. It contains a lot of valuable information, and the material may have saved my life. In my opinion, Lloyd Ney, the founder of PAACT, is a saint. Support groups, regardless of their affiliation, are extremely important sources of information.

If there is one book I would recommend, it is *Cancer Battle Plan* by Anne Frahm, which I mentioned earlier in this book. I read it and immediately felt that I could do this. I could beat cancer. It was a great inspiration to me.

Being a part of the book retreat was an unforgettable experience for Lynne and me. I learned a lot, and I think hearing about all the different therapies and procedures the rest of the guys went through and the feelings I have for each one of them only made me feel more blessed that I am still here. My world has definitely broadened from knowing the nine other men who contributed to this book. I consider them my brothers.

## Some Final Thoughts

As you've no doubt noticed, we all have strong opinions, and we wish to reemphasize they are just that—personal opinions nurtured and strengthened by our own experiences with this disease. We hope that the lessons we've learned will help you to make the decisions best for you. If we could summarize that which is most important to us, here's what we'd say:

- If you are 40 years of age or older, get screened for prostate cancer. You may have to ask your doctor for a DRE and/or a PSA test.
- Early detection (and information) is your best weapon against this disease.
- Don't panic if you are diagnosed. You have time and options.
- Join a support group immediately after your diagnosis—before you make a treatment decision. If there isn't a support group in your area, start one!
- Learn as much as you can about this disease, the treatments, and the side effects—and keep learning. Research is ongoing, and new treatments are always under investigation.
- Learn about complementary therapies.
- Get a second, third, or fourth opinion. Don't stop until you're confident that you're making an informed decision.
- Seek out the most highly skilled physicians that you can. They may or may not be in your local area.
- Form a trusted partnership with your physicians. Talk to them openly and frankly.
- Document all your expenses. Don't accept a no from your insurance company.

Above all, remember that knowledge is the key to empowerment.

## Additional Recommendations from Our "Must Read" List

### From Charlie

*Bragg Toxicless Diet,* Paul C. Bragg, M.D., Patricia Bragg.
*Beating Cancer with Nutrition,* Patrick Quillin, M.D.
*How I Survived Prostate Cancer . . . and So Can You.* James Lewis Jr., Ph.D.
*Cancer Battle Plan.* Anne E. Frahm with David J. Frahm.
*Tissue Cleansing Through Bowel Management.* Bernard Jensen, D.C., Ph.D., Nutritionist.
*Prostate Cancer* (American Cancer Society), David G. Bostwick, M.D., Gregory T. MacLennan, M.D., Thayne R. Larson, M.D.

## 254

$O_2$ *Therapies.* Ed McCabe.
*Healing the Sick.* T. L. Osborn.
*Healing Energy.* Ruth Fishel.
*Don't Sweat the Small Stuff.* Richard Carlson, Ph.D.

### From Virgil

*50 Essential Things to Do When the Doctor Says It's Cancer.* Greg Anderson.
*Prostate Cancer: A Survivor's Guide.* Don Kaltenbach with Tim Richards.
*If You Meet the Buddha on the Road, Kill Him!* Sheldon B. Kopp.
*Man to Man.* Michael Korda.
*How I Survived Prostate Cancer . . . and So Can You,* James Lewis Jr., Ph.D.
*My Prostate and Me.* William Martin.
*Prostate Cancer: Making Survival Decisions.* Sylvan Meyer and Seymour C. Nash.
*Prostate Cancer: A Non-Surgical Perspective.* Dr. Kent Wallner.

### From Manuel

*My Prostate and Me.* William Martin.
*Prostate Cancer: What Every Man and His Family Needs to Know.* David G. Bostwick, M.D., Gregory T. MacLennan, M.D., Thayne R. Larson, M.D.
*Prostate and Cancer: A Family Guide to Diagnosis, Treatment & Survival.* Sheldon Marks, M.D.
*The Scientific American Magazine Special Cancer Edition.* 1995.

### From Derek

*New Guidelines for Surviving Prostate Cancer.* James Lewis Jr., Ph.D., E. Roy Berger, M.D.
*Love, Medicine, and Miracles.* Bernie S. Siegel, M.D.
*Choices in Healing.* Michael Lerner.

*Do not stand*
*at my grave and weep,*
*I am not there. I do not sleep.*
*I am a thousand winds that blow.*
*I am the diamond glints on snow.*
*I am the sunlight*
*on ripened grain.*
*I am the gentle autumn rain.*
*When you awake in the*
*morning's hush*
*I am the soft uplifting rush*
*of quiet birds in circling flight.*
*I am the soft star that*
*shines at night.*
*Do not stand at my grave and cry.*
*I am not there.*
*I did not die.*

*Until we meet again, may God hold you in the palm of his hand.*
(from the Irish blessing)

# *Epilogue*

When I was assigned the task to write a book on prostate cancer, little did I know what I would be getting into, or for that matter, the wonderful people I would come to love. It was clear from the first moments of meeting that we had gathered together a very special group of people—ten men and four women—all intensely committed to this project and to educating the public about prostate cancer.

In the course of writing this book, Paul and Phyllis, Bud, John and Rosalie, Charlie, Virgil, Peter, Manuel and Mary, Bob, Derek, and Don and Lynne taught me, encouraged me, humored me, and helped me understand this disease. With much patience they responded to my many, many requests and questions, did their assigned 'homework,' and carefully proofed my copy. I feel very honored to have worked with all of them—and fortunate that they agreed to work with me.

As I write this, I am painfully aware that we have lost another member of our team. Charlie Russ passed away December 5, 1998. Charlie was one of the first of the group to say yes to this project two years ago. We would spend much time on the phone as he passionately educated me about the issues surrounding this disease. I will never forget our wonderful conversations, his unbridled enthusiasm—and the way he could make a Steinway sing.

Shortly before his death, Charlie told me how difficult a decision it was for him to refrain from further treatment. This was Charlie after all. He had fiercely battled prostate cancer for seven years—never giving up and always researching a new therapy that could help him live longer and better. He knew that he had given this disease everything he had.

Charlie was a champion. He will be buried in the spring of 1999 at the University of Notre Dame.

Finally, I want to say thank you to all the contributors who so generously gave of their time and knowledge. Your honesty and commitment to this project, and compassion for your fellow men and women have produced a uniquely personal book and an unforgettable experience. You are my friends, and I hope that our paths will continue to cross many times in the coming years.

Together we *will* find a cure for prostate cancer.

*N.J.*

# Glossary

**Acid phosphatase**  a substance made in the prostate. Elevated acid phosphatase levels can signal something is wrong with the prostate.

**Adenocarcinoma**  a cancer that develops in the lining or inner surface of an organ. More than 95% of prostate cancers are adenocarcinomas.

**Adjuvant treatment**  treatment that is added to increase effectiveness of a primary therapy.

**Adrenal glands**  two glands located above the kidneys that produce small amounts of the male hormone testosterone as well as other hormones.

**Alkaline phosphatase**  an enzyme produced in the liver and bones that is used to help detect liver or bone metastasis.

**Analog**  a synthetic compound similar to one manufactured by the body. An example is the LHRH (luteinizing hormone-releasing hormone) analog Lupron.

**Androgens**  male hormones, such as testosterone, necessary for the development of the male sex organs and male sexual characteristics such as deep voice and facial hair.

**Androgen independent**  cancer cells that do not require male hormones to grow.

**Androgen receptor sites**  highly specific "locks" in cells that are opened or activated only by androgens, or male hormones, which act as "keys."

**Anemia**  a condition caused by a reduction in the amount of red blood cells produced by the bone marrow. Can be caused by cancer spreading to the bone. Symptoms include feeling tired and weak.

**Aneuploid cells**  cancer cells that contain more chromosomes than normal cells. They tend to be faster growing and more aggressive.

**Antiandrogen (antiandrogen therapy)**  a drug that blocks the activity of an androgen hormone by blocking the androgen receptor sites in target organ cells.

**Antibiotics**  drugs that kill bacteria.

**Antiemetics**  medicines to help control nausea and vomiting. Antiemetics comes from the Greek word *emetikos* which means to vomit.

**Antioxidant**  synthetic or natural substance such as Vitamins A, C, E, believed to help in the prevention of cancer by stopping free radicals from forming.

**Assay**  method of examining or analyzing the presence, absence, or quantity of one or more components of a substance.

**Asymptomatic**  without obvious signs or symptoms of disease. When cancer is in its earliest stages it may develop and grow without symptoms.

**Autologous transfusion**  using a person's own blood for transfusion during surgery.

**Benign**  a growth that is not cancerous.

**Benign prostatic hyperplasia (BPH)**  a noncancerous condition in which the prostate grows and pushes against the urethra and the bladder blocking the flow of urine.

**Bilateral orchiectomy (castration)**  the surgical removal of the testicles.

**Biopsy**  the removal and microscopic examination of a sample of tissue to determine if cancer is present.

**Bladder**  organ in which urine is stored before it is discharged from the body.

**Bladder catheterization**  passage of a catheter into the urinary bladder through the urethra.

**Blood chemistry**  analysis of multiple components in the blood serum including tests to evaluate function of the liver and kidneys, minerals, and cholesterol. Abnormal values can indicate spread of cancer or side effects of treatments.

**Bone scan**  an image that can show disease or trauma to the bones. Doctors inject a radioactive chemical into the bloodstream which goes directly to areas in the bones which may have tumor metastasis or prior injury, such as a previously broken bone.

**Cachexia**  the accelerated weight loss or wasting syndrome suffered by many people with cancer, leaving them weak, malnourished, and emaciated.

**Capsule**  the layer of cells around an organ such as the prostate.

**Castration**  removal of the testicles. See orchiectomy.

**Chemotherapy**  treatment of cancer with certain chemicals that attack and destroy certain types of cancer cells.

**Clinical trial**  use of a new medication or treatment, under strict controls, to see if the new therapy is safe and effective.

**Combination hormonal therapy (CHT)**  the blocking of the effects of testosterone on prostate cancer cells through surgical or chemical castration plus an antiandrogen. Also known as Total Androgen Blockade.

**Computerized axial tomography (CT Scan or CAT scan)**  an x-ray procedure that uses a computer to produce a detailed picture or cross-section of the body. Useful in evaluating soft tissue organs.

**Cryosurgery (cryotherapy)** freezing of the prostate to kill cancer cells through the use of liquid nitrogen probes inserted into the prostate.

**Cystoscope** fiber–optic instrument having a narrow tube with a light at one end. Used to look inside the bladder and urethra.

**Cystoscopy** an examination of the urethra and bladder with a cystoscope.

**Debulk** to reduce the volume of cancer, by surgery, hormone therapy, or chemotherapy.

**Digital rectal exam (DRE)** a procedure in which a physician inserts a gloved finger in the rectum to examine the prostate and surrounding area for any lumps, enlargements or areas of hardness that might indicate the presence of cancer.

**Diploid cells** cancer cells with two sets of chromosomes, or the amount found in normal cells. Tend to be slower growing and less aggressive.

**DNA** vital genetic information ("genetic blueprints") contained in the nucleus of every cell.

**DNA ploidy analysis** an analysis of prostate cancer cells from a biopsy that enables a more accurate determination of the amount of DNA in the cell. The amount of DNA helps determine how fast the cancer cells will grow.

**Drug interaction** any mechanism by which one drug may interact with the action(s) or another drug.

**Edema** swelling caused by the retention or accumulation of fluid in a part of the body.

**Ejaculate** emission of semen at the climax of sexual intercourse.

**Erectile dysfunction** the inability to achieve and maintain an erection sufficient for sexual intercourse.

**Estrogens** female hormones. Oral estrogens, taken as hormonal therapy by men with prostate cancer, reduce testosterone to the castrate range.

**Family physician** primary-care doctor who treats all members of a family.

**Foley catheter** latex or silicone tube inserted into the penis and threaded through the urethra to the bladder. Drains urine from the bladder to an outside collecting bag.

**Free radicals** high energy, unstable chemical substances that cause cell damage, which can lead to the development of cancer.

**Frozen section** a technique in which tissue is removed by biopsy, then frozen, cut into thin slices, and examined under a microscope by a pathologist. Pathologist can usually rapidly examine a frozen section for immediate diagnosis during surgery.

**Gland** structure or organ that produces a substance to be used in another part of the body.

**Gleason score** a method of classifying the grade of cancer by its microscopic appearance. Used to help determine how aggressive the cancer is and how fast it will grow.

**Gynecomastia**  a tender enlargement of the male breasts.

**Hematuria**  blood in the urine.

**Hormonally independent cells**  cancer cells that are not affected by hormones.

**Hormonal therapy**  the use of drugs or surgery to prevent cancer cells from getting the hormones needed to grow. In prostate cancer this means the hormone testosterone and other androgens.

**Hormones**  substances responsible for secondary sex characteristics.

**Hot flashes**  sudden feelings of warmth in the face, neck, upper chest, and back, often with sweating and flushing of the skin. Side effect of some hormonal therapies.

**Hypercalcemia**  a condition caused by too much calcium being released into the bloodstream from the bones. Can be caused by some of the treatments for cancer.

**Immune system**  complicated system of organs, tissues, blood cells, and substances to fight off infections, cancers, and other illnesses.

**Immunotherapy**  treatment by stimulation of the body's own immune system.

**Impotence**  inability to have and maintain an erection suitable for sexual intercourse.

**Incontinence**  inability to hold urine in the bladder. Also called urinary incontinence.

**Informed consent**  permission given by a patient for treatment after learning about and understanding the possible benefits and risks.

**Insurance caps**  the lifetime amount that your policy will cover for a specific illness.

**Interstitial**  within an organ, such as interstitial brachytherapy which is the implanting of radioactive seeds into the prostate to kill cancer.

**Investigational new drug (IND)**  a drug allowed by the FDA to be used in clinical trials but not yet approved for sale to the general public.

**Jewett system (also called Whitmore-Jewett system)**  system of staging cancer to evaluate tumor involvement, lymph note involvement, and whether cancer has spread to other sites or organs. This system is rated A through D.

**Kegel exercises**  pelvic exercises that help to strengthen urinary control.

**Laparoscopic lymphadenectomy**  the removal of pelvic lymph nodes with a laparoscope done through four small incisions in the lower abdominal area.

**LHRH analogs (agonists)**  synthetic compounds of the body's chemical LHRH. These drugs cause the brain to stop stimulating testosterone production.

**Libido**  sex drive

**Localized prostate cancer**   cancer that is confined within the prostate.

**Local recurrence of cancer**   when cancer returns to the prostate or nearby tissue after treatment.

**Luteinizing hormone (LH)**   a chemical signal transmitted by the pituitary. LH tells the testicles to make testosterone.

**Luteinizing hormone-releasing hormone (LHRH)**   a chemical signal made in the brain. LHRH tells the pituitary to make LH.

**Lymphadenectomy**   a procedure in which lymph nodes are taken from your body for purposes of diagnosing or staging cancer.

**Lymphatic system**   network including the lymph nodes, lymph vessels, and lymph fluid; can also be an avenue of spread for cancer cells.

**Lymph nodes**   small bean-shaped structures scattered along the vessels of the lymphatic system. The nodes filter bacteria, viruses, and cancer cells that may travel through the system.

**Magnetic resonance imaging (MRI)**   a painless, noninvasive way of imaging inside the body. Gives three-dimensional views of the body without using x-rays.

**Malignant**   cancerous, with the potential for uncontrolled growth and spread.

**Margin negative**   condition where cancer cells are not found on the edges of tissue that has been cut out during surgery. A negative margin indicates that there's a good chance all of the cancerous tissue was removed.

**Margin positive**   condition in which cancer cells are found at the cut edge of tissue removed during surgery. A positive margin indicates that it's not certain if the surgeon was able to cut out all the cancer.

**Medical oncologist**   a doctor with special training in the diagnosis, treatment, and evaluation of cancer and in the use of drugs for chemotherapy and hormone therapy to treat cancer. He or she has also had training in internal medicine. A medical oncologist can follow you concurrently with your urologist.

**Metastasis**   the spread of cancer cells from one part of the body (the main tumor site) to other organs or tissues through the lymphatic or blood systems. (metastases, *pl.*, metastatic, *adj.*)

**Nerve sparing technique**   a surgical technique during a radical prostatectomy where one or both of the neurovascular bundles controlling erections are spared. The utilization of this procedure depends on the extent of the cancer.

**Nocturia**   a condition where an individual must get up several times during the night to urinate.

**Oncology**   the branch of medical science dealing with cancer.

**Oncology nurse**   a nurse who specializes in the care of persons with cancer. Oncology nurses take an active role in pain and symptom management.

**Orchiectomy (castration)**  the surgical removal of the testicles.

**Orgasm**  the climax of sexual intercourse.

**Outpatient**  describes a surgery or treatment that does not require an overnight stay in the hospital.

**Palliative care/treatment**  therapy that relieves symptoms such as pain, but does not alter the course of the disease. Its primary purpose is to improve the quality of life.

**Palpable**  can be felt. Palpable cancer in the prostate means there's a lump or nodule that a doctor's gloved finger can feel during a digital rectal exam (DRE).

**Pathologist**  a doctor who specializes in the diagnosis of disease by studying cells and tissues removed from the body.

**Pathologic fracture**  bones that have broken due to brittleness caused by the invasion of cancer. Men with metastatic prostate cancer are susceptible to broken bones.

**PDQ**  a database available to physicians and patients on the latest information on standard treatments and ongoing clinical trials for each type and stage of cancer.

**Penile**  relating to the penis.

**Penile implants**  bendable, inflatable, or mechanical prostheses that enable an impotent man to have erections.

**Perineal prostatectomy**  an operation to remove the prostate gland from an opening between the scrotum and the anus.

**Perineum**  the area between the scrotum and the anus.

**Placebo**  a substance that has no real therapeutic pharmacological value such as a sugar pill—instead of actual medicine. Occasionally used in research studies in which a new medication is being studied, but rarely used in clinical studies for cancer.

**Placebo effect**  a phenomenon that happens in medical studies, in which patients taking a placebo have an inexplicable improvement in symptoms.

**Ploidy status**  the genetic status of cancer cells; similar to the grade.

**Poorly-differentiated**  cancer cells that have poorly defined borders. Considered high-grade and aggressive cancer that spreads rapidly.

**Positive biopsy**  the detection of cancer in a biopsy.

**Primary tumor**  the site where a malignancy starts.

**Prognosis**  a prediction of the course of the disease and the future prospects for survival and recovery of the patient.

**Prostate**  a muscular, walnut-shaped gland about an inch and a half long that sits directly below the bladder.

**Prostatectomy**  the surgical removal of all or part of the prostate.

**Prostatic specific antigen (PSA)**  an enzyme produced by the prostate. PSA levels, measured by a simple blood test, are used to help detect and monitor prostate cancer.

**Prosthesis**   artificial replacement for part of the body that is either missing or not functioning properly.

**PSA velocity**   PSA's rate of change.

**Radiation therapy**   treatment using x-rays to destroy cancerous tissues.

**Radiation oncologist**   a doctor who specializes in the use of radiation to treat cancer. Radiation may be used to treat early or advanced prostate cancer. In advanced prostate cancer, it is frequently used for palliative care. A radiation oncologist can follow you concurrently with your urologist.

**Radical prostatectomy**   surgery to remove the prostate and surrounding tissues and structures, including the seminal vesicles, to eliminate cancer.

**Receptors**   highly specific "locks" in cells that are opened or activated only by certain hormones or chemical signals, which act as "keys."

**Recurrence**   return of a disease.

**Refractory**   a term commonly used to describe a situation where the disease is no longer controlled by current therapy.

**Relative survival rates**   the differences in survival between men who are alive and living with the disease and men who don't have prostate cancer. That means that 85% of men diagnosed with prostate cancer will survive for at least five years compared to 100% of men who don't have the disease, when corrected for deaths from other causes.

**Remission**   complete or partial disappearance of the signs and symptoms of disease in response to treatment. Can be temporary or permanent.

**Resect**   to surgically remove, or cut out.

**Retropubic prostatectomy**   surgery to remove the prostate gland and seminal vesicles through the lower abdomen.

**Scrotum**   sac that holds the testicles.

**Secondary tumor**   tumor created by cells which have broken away from the primary tumor and traveled to another part of the body.

**Semen**   the fluid that transports sperm.

**Seminal vesicles**   glands at the base of the bladder that produce fluid and nutrients for semen.

**Small-cell carcinoma**   a type of prostate cancer. Cells in these tumors are similar to other small-cell cancers (the lung, for example), and respond to the same kinds of chemotherapy drugs used to treat these tumors.

**Sphincter**   a bundle of muscles surrounding a tubular organ and controlling passage of fluid, such as the urinary sphincter.

**Staging**   determining the extent of a cancer; if it's still confined to the prostate, how big it is, or how far it has spread. The stage of prostate cancer helps to determine the appropriate therapy. The two main systems for staging prostate cancer are the Whitmore-Jewett and the TNM system.

**Stents**   tubes that are implanted and left in place to allow drainage from one place to another. In the case of BPH, they're placed in the urethra to ease obstructed urinary flow.

**Stress incontinence**   the leakage of urine during certain activities such as running or golf.

**Stricture**   blockage caused by scar tissue. Can squeeze down on a channel such as the urethra.

**Subcapsular orchiectomy**   surgical removal of the testicles where the surgeon opens the lining to the testicles, empties the contents of each testicle, and then closes the lining. The empty shell is placed back inside the scrotum to maintain appearance.

**Suprapubic**   above the pubic bone. In a suprapubic prostatectomy, the surgeon reaches the prostate by making an incision in the lower abdomen, then goes through the bladder to reach the prostate.

**Surgical margins**   determined when pathologists look at the edges of tissue that has been cut out during surgery. If cancer cells are not found on these edges, then the margin is negative, indicating there's a good chance all of the cancerous tissue was removed. If cancer cells are found, then the margin is positive, indicating that it's not certain if the surgeon was able to cut out all the cancer.

**Systemic**   throughout the body.

**Testicles**   a man's reproductive organs inside the scrotum. They produce sperm, testosterone, and other sex hormones.

**Testosterone**   a male sex hormone, or androgen, produced by the testicles. It is associated with growth and activity of the prostate. Lowering testosterone levels is a major goal of hormonal therapy to treat prostate cancer.

**Tetraploid cells**   cancer cells that contain more chromosomes than normal cells. Tend to be faster growing and more aggressive.

**TNM (Tumor Node Metastasis)**   international staging of cancer determined by combining information about the extent of the tumor in the prostate gland, the involvement of the lymph nodes, and whether it has metastasized to other areas or organs.

**Total androgen blockade**   see Combination Hormonal Therapy (CHT).

**Transperineal**   through the perineum, the area between the scrotum and the anus.

**Transrectal**   through the rectum.

**Transrectal ultrasound of the prostate (TRUS/P)**   A test using sound wave echoes to create an image of an organ or gland to visually inspect it for abnormal conditions. It is also extremely useful for guidance of needle biopsies of the prostate, and guiding the nitrogen probes in cryosurgery.

**Transurethral**   through the urethra.

**Transurethral incision of the prostate (TUIP)**   a surgical technique for treating BPH on individuals with small prostates.

**Transurethral needle ablation (TUNA)**   a procedure used to treat BPH. Radio frequency energy is conducted through tiny needles, inserted directly into prostate tissue via a catheter.

**Transurethral resection of the prostate (TUR or TURP)**  a surgical procedure used to treat BPH. A fiber–optic instrument is placed up the urethra, allowing the surgeon to see prostate tissue that is blocking urinary flow. Portions of the prostate are removed in fragments by the instrument, through the urethra. Also called the "Roto-Rooter" procedure.

**Tumor flare**  when LHRH agonists may temporarily stimulate tumor growth and symptoms. To prevent this, doctors usually recommend taking an antiandrogen every eight hours beginning at least two days before the first Lupron shot or Zoladex injection.

**Ultrasound**  painless, noninvasive use of high-frequency sound waves to produce an image or photograph of a tissue or organ.

**Ureter**  the tube that carries urine from each kidney to the bladder.

**Urethra**  the tube that carries urine from the bladder and fluid from the prostate through the penis to the outside of the body.

**Urinary retention**  inability to urinate, with the bladder filling up with urine.

**Urinary tract obstruction**  a blockage of the urinary tract causing difficulty in urinating, or not being able to urinate at all. Can be the result of cancer spreading extensively to the bladder.

**Urologist**  a doctor who specializes in the diagnoses and treatment of diseases of the urinary tracts of men and women and the genital organs of men. Urologists are surgeons who perform the operations for prostate cancer. Urologists may also administer hormonal therapy, and/or follow you concurrently with your oncologist.

**Vascular**  involving blood vessels.

**Vas deferens**  tiny muscular tube that transports sperm from the testicles to the prostate gland.

**Vasectomy**  a surgical procedure to make a man sterile by cutting the vas deferens so that sperm can no longer pass through into the semen.

**Venous**  relating to the veins.

**Venous leak**  a common cause of erection problems. The arteries fill the penis with blood, producing a partial erection, but the veins don't clamp down to keep the blood trapped inside the penis.

**Viaticals**  involves the cash sale of your life insurance policy to a third party. People who choose a viatical settlement generally receive about 60% or more of the face value of their policy immediately in return for signing over the benefits. Generally for people who have less than 24 months to live.

**Well-differentiated**  cancer cells with clearly defined borders and clear centers. Considered to be low-grade and less aggressive.